HOW DOCTORS THINK

HOW DOCTORS THINK

CLINICAL JUDGMENT AND THE PRACTICE
OF MEDICINE

Kathryn Montgomery

OXFORD

UNIVERSITY PRESS

2006

OXFORD
UNIVERSITY PRESS

Oxford University Press, Inc., publishes works that further
Oxford University's objective of excellence
in research, scholarship, and education.

Oxford   New York
Auckland   Cape Town   Dar es Salaam   Hong Kong   Karachi
Kuala Lumpur   Madrid   Melbourne   Mexico City   Nairobi
New Delhi   Shanghai   Taipei   Toronto

With offices in
Argentina   Austria   Brazil   Chile   Czech Republic   France   Greece
Guatemala   Hungary   Italy   Japan   Poland   Portugal   Singapore
South Korea   Switzerland   Thailand   Turkey   Ukraine   Vietnam

Copyright © 2006 by Oxford University Press, Inc.

Published by Oxford University Press, Inc.
198 Madison Avenue, New York, New York 10016
www.oup.com
Oxford is a registered trademark of Oxford University Press

CIP data available from the Library of Congress
ISBN-13 978-0-19-518712-0
ISBN 0-19-518712-1

3 5 7 9 8 6 4 2

Printed in the United States of America
on acid-free paper

To Anne, Ellen, Eric, Will, Jesse, Paul, Sallyann, Megan, Samantha, Ben, Anna, Lisa, Aaron, Jacob, Elijah, Debra, Michael, Hunter, Hannah, Beth, and Tom—for whom I'm thankful all year round.

ACKNOWLEDGMENTS

OVER THE LAST decade, usefully critical audiences have commented on various arguments in this book, and editors—kindly, impatiently, or both—have nudged early versions of several chapters into print. My gratitude to them is acknowledged in the notes to each. Here I want to record more general, comprehensive thanks. Because my ideas about the relation of medicine to science took shape during an earlier study of narrative in clinical teaching, research, and patient care, many of my debts are old ones. Edmund Pellegrino first suggested to me that an education in literature might have advantages for understanding medicine. I remain grateful to the National Science Foundation, which knew that medicine is not a science but risked an Ethics and Values in Science and Technology grant for that earlier project, and to the American Council of Learned Societies, whose polysemous initials (in medicine, they stand for Advanced Cardiac Life Support) suggest the value of its year's support. My interest in the representation of clinical knowledge goes back to my 1981 National Endowment for the Humanities summer seminar, "The Power of the Healer," and I remember often, even at this late date, the people who attended and those who joined me in teaching. I am still grateful to my colleagues at the University of Rochester who were willing to teach me what I needed to know about ethnography, epistemology, and clinical medicine and unfailingly asked hard questions about what a literary scholar was doing in a place like a medical school.

Since that time I have incurred a new, long list of debts. The first is to Tod Chambers, with whom I have taught and argued for more than a decade at Northwestern, to James F. Bresnahan, S. J., who began the medical humanities and bioethics program there and welcomed me as his successor, and to my colleagues: Peter Angelos, Hillel Braude, Jacqueline Cameron, Rowland Chang, Raymond Curry, Jorge Daaboul, Joel Frader, Lester Friedman, Warren Furey, Robert Golub, Philip Greenland, Robert Hirschtick, Joshua Hauser, Kristi Kirschner, Myria Knox, Ellen LeVee, John Merrill, Maureen Brady Moran,

Scott Moses, David Neely, Kathy Johnson Neely, Douglas Reifler, Henry Ruder, John Sanders, Carol Schilling, Katie Watson, the late Bob Winter, and the Work-in-Progress Group of the Medical Humanities and Bioethics Program. For sixteen years the Chicago Narrative and Medicine Reading Group has provided good arguments and good things to read, thanks to its convener, Suzanne Poirier, and, among others, William J. Donnelly, George Karnezis, Mary Jeanne Larrabee, Ann Folwell Stanford, Barbara Sharf, and Patrick Staunton.

Drafts of chapters or the whole manuscript were read by Stephen Adams, James F. Bresnahan, S.J., Howard Brody, Tod Chambers, Julia Connelly, Raymond H. Curry, Sandra Bain Cushman, Bill Donnelly, Carl Elliott, Ruth Freeman, Ross Kessel, Kristi Kirschner, Heinz Kuehn, Lewis Landsberg, John Merrill, David Morris, Phebe Kirkland, Eliezer Margolis, Karen Pralinsky, Douglas Reifler, Teresa Savage, Katie Watson, Mark Waymack, and the fastest, best editor in the East, Ellen Key Harris-Braun. She and Joan Boomsma, Catherine Caldicott, Jacqueline Cameron, Rowland Chang, Rita Charon, Julia Connelly, Deb DeRosa, Roger Dunteman, the late Rita Serrins Glazer, Lowell Goldstein, Joseph Hart, Anne Montgomery Hunter, Paul Hunter, John Merrill, Beth Montgomery, Sherwin Nuland, Suzanne Poirier, Risha O'Connor Raven, Douglas Reifler, Richard Schuster, Barbara Sharf, Michael Woodruff, and the much missed Beth Fine Kaplan provided details that are not acknowledged in the notes. Michael Morgan sent me books on case-based reasoning from Morgan-Kaufmann Publishers, and Debra Hunter sent Donald Schön's from Jossey-Bass. Shannon Matthews at the University of Chicago bookstore fixed my Macintosh one rainy summer afternoon; Macario Flores at Northwestern's Feinberg Computer Lab generously provided technical support, and Eric Harris-Braun always answered computer questions in record time. Susan Weissman, Doug, Katherine, and Erin Reifler offered me shelter when the revision process most needed it. Eric Cassell, who wrote years ago to say he liked *Doctors' Stories* but "You need more steel," has been one of my imagined readers. So, too, has Lewis White Beck, who died in 1997 but remains the Kantian I wanted most to persuade. For many helpful discussions and for their company on various adventures I am especially grateful to Julia Connelly and Susan Squier.

Last are the immeasurable debts: first, to students who over the years have talked to me so generously about the process of becoming a physician and to colleagues who have been willing to reflect on the puzzles and pleasures of taking care of patients; and, finally, to Barbara Burtness, Cecile Carson, Rita Charon, Carol Staugaard Hahn, Paul LoGerfo, and Constance Park, skilled clinicians who do their best so well.

CONTENTS

‿⸒

HOW DOCTORS THINK

INTRODUCTION

⌐⌐

Rationality in an Uncertain Practice

It does not do harm to the mystery to know a little about it.

—RICHARD FEYNMAN

THIS BOOK IS about clinical judgment: why it is essential to medical practice even in a highly scientific, technologized era, how it works in that practice, some of the odd ways it is taught, and the consequences of ignoring it in favor of the assumption that medicine is itself a science.

There is no question that medicine is scientific or that the benefits of biomedicine are enormous. Once doomed lives are now routinely saved, and the sense of human possibility has been profoundly altered. Yet medicine is not itself a science. Despite its reliance on a well-stocked fund of scientific knowledge and its use of technology, it is still a practice: the care of sick people and the prevention of disease. The recent emphasis on evidence-based medicine grounds that practice more firmly in clinical research and aims to refine and extend clinical judgment, but it will not alter the character of medicine or its rationality. Physicians draw on their diagnostic skills and clinical experience as well as scientific information and clinical research when they exercise clinical judgment. Bodies are regarded as rule-governed entities and diseases as invading forces or guerrillas biding their time. But neither is true. Patients with the same diagnosis can differ unpredictably, and maladies, even those firmly identified with bacteria or tumors or genetic mutations, are never quite *things*. Thus, although scientific and technological advances refine clinical problems and provide solutions, physicians still work in situations of inescapable uncertainty. New diseases like human immunodeficiency virus (HIV) or severe acute respiratory syndrome (SARS) are the extreme examples, but everyday cases are uncertain, too. Useful information is available in overwhelming quantities, and physicians have the daily task of sorting through it and deciding how some part applies to an individual patient in a given circumstance.

How does a physician know? The question scarcely bears thinking about, for being ill and depending on a doctor's advice and treatment can be terrifying even when life is not at stake. For centuries physicians and their methods were objects of satire in novels and plays, paintings and prints: think of Molière's *Le Malade Imaginaire* or Fielding's *Tom Jones* or Hogarth's *Harlot's Progress*. Not until early in the twentieth century did a sick person have a better-than-even chance of benefiting from consulting a physician. Today, when diagnosis and treatment are based on scientific research, seeking medical help is an enormously improved but still uncertain quest.[1] That uncertainty is ritualized, professionalized, and then for the most part ignored by both the patients who seek help and the physicians who must act on their behalf.[2]

Scientific information reduces but does not eliminate medicine's uncertainty. As a result, medical education is crammed to overflowing with what is known, yet the long clinical apprenticeship that is its essence prepares physicians to act in uncertain circumstances. Physicians must learn not only what course of action will be most likely to benefit the patient (even when the choices are not good ones) but also what to do when information is conflicting or unavailable. For this reason, medical education is a moral as well as an intellectual education: experiential, behavioral, and in important ways covert.[3] It is also hierarchical, ritualized, and characterized by paradoxes and contradictions that foster habits of skepticism and thoroughness. Physicians are trained to aim for maximal certainty. But because the unexpected cannot be excluded, they are also taught to be exquisitely aware of anomaly. Then, as if to cement confidence in this uncertain, paradox-laden, judgment-dependent practice, their work is described—despite the evidence—as an old-fashioned, positivist, Newtonian science. Instead, it is a rational, science-using practice that idealizes a simplified, old-fashioned vision of science.

The claim that medicine is a science, especially in an outdated sense of the word, does not begin to do the profession justice. Medicine's simplified idea of science is not the creative social enterprise that sociologists and philosophers of science have described over the last 30 years, but rather the realist vision of physical certainty taught in grade school and presented in the media. With its invariable replicability and law-like precision, this view of science is a matter of simple logic with readily deduced details and rule-governed consequences. What characterizes the care of patients, however, is contingency. It requires practical reasoning, or *phronesis*, which Aristotle described as the flexible, interpretive capacity that enables moral reasoners (and the physicians and navigators that he compares with them) to determine the best action to take when knowledge depends on circumstance.[4] Today we might add engineers and meteorologists and even Xerox copier technicians to the list.[5] In medicine that interpretive capacity is clinical judgment, and this book attempts to describe that intelligence: how it differs from the rationality of science that medicine idealizes, how it displaces or contravenes science in practice, how it is taught, and how recognizing its importance might reduce some of the adverse side effects of the belief that medicine is itself a science.

Two and half millennia of scientific discovery—including the advances of the last two and half decades—have not altered medicine's practical rationality. No matter how solid the science or how precise the technology that physicians use, clinical medicine remains an interpretive practice. Medicine's success relies on the physicians' capacity for clinical judgment. It is neither a science nor a technical skill (although it puts both to use) but the ability to work out how general rules—scientific principles, clinical guidelines—apply to one particular patient. This is—to use Aristotle's word—*phronesis*, or practical reasoning.[6] It enables physicians to combine scientific information, clinical skill, and collective experience with similar patients to make sense of the particulars of one patient's illness and to determine the best action to take to cure or alleviate it. Although young residents often ridicule appeals to clinical judgment as the last refuge of an out-of-date physician, good clinical judgment nevertheless is the goal of medical education and the ideal of every physician's practice.

This book is an account of how doctors think: their exercise of clinical judgment as they work out what is best to do for a particular patient. It looks at the odd contradictions involved in clinical medicine's misrepresentation as a science and at the tension-filled clinical education that transforms students of science into reliable practical reasoners. It explores the way clinical judgment works in diagnosis and therapy and how it narrows and simplifies the idea of cause. It considers why clinical judgment, despite being the goal of medical education and the ideal of practice, is ignored in favor of the misdescription of medicine as a science—and some of the reasons for that neglect. Understanding the nature of clinical practice goes a good way toward explaining the reasons for medicine's misrepresentation of its work. The widespread misdescription of medicine as a science and the failure to appreciate its chief virtue, clinical judgment or phronesis, amount to a visual field defect in the understanding of medicine.[7] In medical-philosophical terms, the misunderstanding of clinical reasoning is an epistemological *scotoma*, a blindness of which the knower is unaware. I want to describe that blindness (and, especially, the profession's blindness to it) and to try to explain why it persists.

My curiosity has been all the stronger because misunderstanding the epistemology of medicine—how doctors know what they know—has damaging consequences for patients, for the profession of medicine, and for physicians themselves. The assumption that medicine is a science—a positivist what-you-see-is-what-there-is representation of the physical world—passes almost unexamined by physicians, patients, and society as a whole. The costs are great. It has led to a harsh, often brutal education, unnecessarily impersonal clinical practice, dissatisfied patients, and disheartened physicians.[8] In the United States, where the idea of medicine as a science is perhaps strongest, the misrepresentation of how physicians think and work contributes to the failure to provide basic health care to citizens and to a confusion of bad outcome with malpractice that has resulted in an epidemic of debilitating lawsuits. Although there are understandable reasons for the claim that medicine is a science and for the assumption that physicians reason like positivist scientists, I argue instead for an examination of medicine's rationality in practice and for the importance of clinical judgment as its characteristic intellectual virtue, a rational capacity that human beings necessarily employ in uncertain circumstances. Like history or evolutionary biology, clinical medicine is fated to be a retrospective, narrative investigation and not a Newtonian or Galilean science. Aristotle's pronouncement that there can be no science of individuals suggests the difficult, counterbalancing, often paradoxical nature of the work physicians are called to do.[9] In undertaking the care of a patient, physicians—however scientific they may be—are not engaged in a quantifiable science but in a rational, interpretive practice.

This account of medicine is that of an outsider, a sort of licensed trespasser in clinical territory. While it might seem inevitable that someone with a Ph.D. in English literature teaching in a medical school would wonder about physicians' thinking and the relative importance of science in that process, my curiosity about medical epistemology began while I still taught undergraduates. When in the 1970s Morehouse College excused Advanced Placement students from the introductory literature course but held fast to its requirement for freshman English, several faculty members devised honors courses in composition and research. My course, "The Evolution of the Idea of Evolution," grew out of a lifelong fascination with science, the history of science, and the ways human beings make sense of perception and experience. These interests had propelled me into the study of literature, where at the intersection of language and culture (or of writer and reader) the problems of representation and interpretation were for me most compelling of all. The course began with Shakespeare, Milton, and Pope and their accounts of humanity's relation to the rest of creation in the "great chain of being" and then focused on *The Voyage of the Beagle* and the science known to Darwin from Adam Smith, Erasmus Darwin, and Lamarck to Ricardo Malthus and Charles Lyell. Students' research projects ranged through the theories of Alfred Russel Wallace and social Darwinism to missing-link racism in American anthropology. Although I hadn't planned this part, the students who signed up were bright biology and chemistry majors hoping to go to medical school. I loved the course and what the students made of it. Soon I was writing letters of recommendation to medical schools, and when my colleagues began planning a new medical school, I was invited to join them.

Well before the medical school at Morehouse opened, I learned the first dispiriting lesson about medical education. My students returned at homecoming or Thanksgiving from their first few months of medical school looking, as the pediatrician Henry K. Silver later described another group of first-year students, like abused children.[10] What had happened? They left smart and diligent, equally devoted to science and success, and sustained more often than not by religious faith. As medical students, they had achieved the almost inalienable first step toward physicianhood, but they were suffering nonetheless. Racial isolation at still very white northern schools was not the primary cause; those who had gone to Howard or Meharry looked just as lackluster and embattled. Years later, at my second medical school, a student nearing the end of the first year in the old, Flexnerian curriculum described the condition: "I'm not learning science," he said dully. "I'm not even learning facts anymore; I'm just learning *things*."

Since that time, much of medical education has undergone real reform.[11] Medical students are now taught separately from biology graduate students. Lecture time has been reduced to merely two or three times that found in the rest of university education. Medical humanities, bioethics, communication skills, medical decision-making, and problem-based learning have refocused the first two years (to varying degrees) on doctoring. Still, for more than two decades, I have puzzled over medicine's relationship to science and the ways academic medicine moderates and counteracts its claim to be a science without ever relinquishing or openly questioning it. How do college students become physicians and what part does scientific knowledge play in the process?

When I moved in 1980 to the University of Rochester, the chance to observe clinicians reflecting on their work led me to extend those questions from education to practice: how do physicians use science? How do good clinicians know what they know, and how is clinical judgment fostered and refined? Clinical clerkships and residency programs proclaim what are understood to be medicine's scientific values; yet at the same time they use long-established clinical and pedagogical methods that bear a contradictory relation to that scientific ideal. The interpretive question this posed for me was unavoidable: What was going on here? For a literary scholar teaching in a medical school, the answer began with discovering the pervasive presence of narrative in clinical practice,[12] but medicine's case-based narrative method is only one facet of the profession's odd relationship to science. Clinical medicine is filled with unexamined paradoxes and contradictions. The frequently expressed suspicion of anecdote that accompanies medicine's reliance on case narrative for its organization and transmission of knowledge is only the most obvious. This book describes a number of others. The overarching oddity is that medicine's ideal of positivist science exists right alongside its use of a flexible, interpretive, ineradicably practical rationality. Beyond the supreme serviceability of biomedical science as a source of information, it is a screen for clinical behavior that, while profoundly unlike what might be expected from the idealization of science, is nevertheless wholly rational in its method and moral in its aim. Why, I wondered, did my colleagues, who are formidably intelligent and experienced clinicians, find it essential to misdescribe (if never quite misunderstand) the rational process by which they work?

This book attempts to answer that question. The first three chapters describe the nature of medicine as a practice and the oddity of the claim that it is (or soon will be) a science. Chapter 1 is an account of the demand for certainty in medicine, a need that runs up against the limits of physicians' practical knowledge. Chapter 2 argues that clinical medicine is neither a science nor art but practical reasoning, an account that takes into consideration the uncertainties inherent in the physician's task of diagnosing and treating sick people. Chapter 3 describes the narrative rationality essential to the exercise of clinical judgment in the absence of certain knowledge of the individual case.

Part II explores the oddities of causal reasoning in clinical medicine and illustrates the ways clinical practice circumvents what might be expected of a science. Chapter 4 compares clinical causality with the idea of science that medicine customarily appeals to and finds that it more closely resembles narrative-based investigation in the social sciences. Chapter 5 argues that medicine's idealization of linear causality fits its goal of diagnosing and treating patients but not the reality of its practice. Chapter 6 addresses the tension in medical practice between scientific generalization and particular details, a tension inherent in practical rationality, and describes the place of evidence-based medicine in clinical practice.

Part III focuses on clinical education and the ways students and residents are encouraged to think outside the box of positivist science, even as that vision of science is held up as medicine's ideal. Chapter 7 looks at the way informal—and contradictory—rules are used to guide clinical judgment. The counterweighted maxims that constitute a theory of clinical knowing are described in chapter 8 as the "bottom-up," practical expression of the tension between generalizable scientific knowledge and the particular knowledge demanded of an interpretive clinical practice. Chapter 9 uses seating patterns in three hospital conferences to argue that the apparently trivial decision about where to sit tests and rewards clinical medicine's hierarchy of knowledge, skill, and experience.

Part IV imagines the benefits of a richer, more complex understanding of clinical medicine and its rationality: for physicians themselves, for society, and for patients and their families. Chapter 10 considers how medicine's claim to be a science is used by physicians in the internalization of professional attitudes and as a defense against the suffering of patients. Chapter 11 goes out on a limb to argue that the scientific aspirations of medical practice have occluded its social ones and left a deficit that has physicians (at least sometimes) longing to regard patients as friends. Chapter 12 argues that clinical practice, and not a simplistic idea of science, is the source of attitudes and values essential to medicine. Understanding medicine as a practice that focuses on care of patients serves patients and physicians far better.

Caveat Lector

As the reader will have already noticed, I use the word "science" in the narrow, old-fashioned, positivist sense borrowed from my clinical colleagues. This is Newton's science: science as the explanation of how things work, how they really are. It gives us the facts, which are understood to be certain, replicable, dependable. Science in this sense is an egregious straw man, but a straw man with very powerful legs. The positivist idea of science—science as the uninflected representation of reality—pervades our culture. It has a strong presence in education, the news media, and the arts. Elementary schools introduce science as a realist and value-neutral endeavor, and most high school courses do little to alter the idea. In the media, journalists not only use "science" in this simplistic way but take it for granted in reporting on medicine: cost containment, technological breakthroughs, malpractice, and, especially, new therapies. Perhaps most important, the idea of medicine as a science is the desperate assumption of patients, including, I suspect, physicians, scientists, and philosophers of medicine when they are ill. Just as the most convinced Copernican among us speaks of the sun rising and setting, so when we or those we love are ill, we find the body to be palpably, painfully real beyond all social construction. Then the body seems best known through science. No wonder that in practice physicians think of medicine as an exact and unmediated representation of reality.

Two other cautions are called for. First, this book is not about nurses—although they too are clinicians, and especially in hospitals, clinical medicine also belongs to them. As a feminist, I admire the discipline's commitment to professionalization and broad scholarship as well as to the care of patients. As a humanist, however, I worry when nursing adopts medicine's scientism. I hope that describing what I know about physicians and their work will contribute to the growing reliance on health-care teams and to the considered autonomy of nurse-practitioners and midwives.

Second, this book is not a sociological study. Rather, it is an extended essay on the nature of medicine and medical education, especially the theory and practice of teachers of clinical medicine. It examines descriptions of medicine and their manifestation in a range of places: literary texts, commencement speeches, habits of phrase, professional rituals, and pedagogical strategies. I have focused especially on the institutional expressions of medicine's goals: the way students and residents are taught that medicine *ought* to be practiced, the way it is idealized in academic medicine. There, in tertiary-care medical centers, is the full panoply of Western medicine: the best and the brightest, standards at their highest, peer review at its sharpest, and assumptions most open to scrutiny.

PART I

Medicine as a Practice

CHAPTER ONE

⌒

Medicine and the Limits of Knowledge

Every living thought represents a gesture made toward
the world, an attitude taken to some practical
situation in which we are implicated.

—JOHN DEWEY

I SET OUT to write a book about clinical judgment: how, given the uncertainty
of its knowledge, medicine is taught and practiced and how its identification
with science affects both patients and physicians. Before I was well into it,
my 28-year-old daughter found a breast lump and had an excisional biopsy.

Physical symptoms are read narratively, contextually, and interpreted in
cultural systems. A physician's diagnosis is a plot summary of a socially
constructed pathophysiological sequence of events. The lump is there. It
is a sign, caught *in medias res*, a clue to a natural history that is unfolding.
Science describes and explains it and determines what can be done about
it. But the importance of that lump, the acts its discovery entails, and what
those acts will mean are social and cultural matters. Although for turn-of-
the-millennium North Americans, culture is shaped by—of a piece with—
Western scientific medicine, within that culture, as Lynn Payer pointed out,
there are significant national variants. The French like breasts, she observed,
and not surprisingly, surgeons in France regularly performed lumpectomies
long before the English and Americans, who like randomized clinical trials.[1] Is
there a fixed, invariant truth about breast cancer and its treatment, a reality that
has nothing to do with culture? Certainly there are scientific facts, refinements
in knowledge, improvements in care. Mastectomy is no longer the automatic
treatment regardless of tumor and breast size. But women in the United States

who 20 years ago were led to have modified radical mastectomies rather than lumpectomies were not duped by their surgeons. Then everyone—patients, surgeons, families—felt more secure trading breasts for what they were convinced was a higher degree of certainty: "They think they got it all." American medicine moved very slowly to investigate the alternatives because the choice was posed as a matter of life or death.[2]

"Invasive ductal carcinoma, moderately differentiated . . ." a pathology lab in Beijing and New York City might both report. But would it be the same? Breast cancer is not common there. Do the Chinese like breasts? One imagines that the meaning of breast cancer in that half of the world might have more to do with maternity and women's social citizenship than sex and the self. The therapy might differ—if not the primary treatment, then the treatment of side effects. The United States has "the best medicine in the world." But, just as U.S. surgeons adopted the German practice of giving valium preoperatively (once it was clear the benefits went beyond calming the patient to lessening the measurable side effects of surgery), might the Chinese know something that U.S. medicine could usefully borrow?

Millions of woman-hours are spent anguishing over the possibility of breast cancer, lump or no lump. Mammograms are never truly routine, even for women fortunate enough to afford periodic screening. Some manage to stay busy until the report is in, even busy enough to neglect to call to be sure the results are negative. But for many the test is a final exam that poses ultimate questions about the relation of self and body, about death and the meaning of life. The obvious answers to these questions are answers in the aggregate. They are common knowledge: we are embodied selves in a strongly gendered, body-conscious society, and those bodies—we ourselves—will die. A mammogram suggests that the ultimate questions also have particular answers and that it may be time to work them out in our own lives. A biopsy leads us to discover, like Tolstoy's Ivan Ilych, that the syllogism ending "Caius is mortal" could just as easily be written with our own name.

When the results are normal, we go back to normal too. We are reimmersed in our ordinary lives and their more immediate concerns.

I wanted to shield my daughter from all this. She was only 28, married not quite a year, absorbed in interesting work. I quoted her the statistics for lumps, the age-weighted probabilities. If not quite negligible, they are minuscule. And besides, this happens. "Large-breasted women often have lumps," I said, putting it in the big, epidemiological picture. I didn't want her to have both a suspicious lump and a mother who teaches in a medical school alarmed about it.

The night before the biopsy I dreamed she lay inert and faded in a hospital bed. I sang to her; but she was too sick to bear it and shook her head weakly. Awake, I understood it as a dream about her younger sister, just out of college and on her own, and the interesting problem of being a good mother to adult daughters. Don't infantilize, I decided it meant.

Two days later the surgeon left a message on her answering machine: he'd call her the next day. But what time? "He could at least have said the report was okay," she said.

I had spent the last 20 years puzzling out what doctors do, and I summoned up a narrative into which his nonmessage fit. "He needs to make you a speech, wants to be sure you go on following these up," I said. "Besides someone probably once told him surgeons shouldn't communicate by answering machine."

She called the next day: "It's not a fibroadenoma. It's real cancer."

My perspective on medicine has changed since then. Although some of what I knew about medicine and the uncertainty of its knowledge was helpful, much of it I completely forgot. Friends were the real help—some in medicine, some out, some licensed trespassers like me. The ground of ordinary life opened up, and I fell through to the breast cancer world, an alternate reality. Colleagues appeared at my door and on my computer screen to talk about their wives, their sisters, themselves. On the sidewalk of my very urban campus, people passing asked with a special emphasis, "How are you?" or waved crossed fingers from the other side of the street. They meant breast cancer; all references were to breast cancer. It was October, breast cancer month, and statistics were everywhere.

Young women don't do well. Their cancers are as lively and energetic as they are. Most are estrogen-receptor negative, which means that tamoxifen—the only therapy that, if not quite benign, is at least not dangerous in itself—for them is useless. And if a devout agnostic pleads with fate that bone and brain scan be clean, that the lymph nodes that surgeons continue to remove be cancer-free, and that plea is granted, then how can she not be grateful for the best odds a 28-year-old can have? Stage I: a 75% five-year disease-free survival rate, improved by chemotherapy to 82%. I rejoiced. I am thankful nonstop.

Still, 82% is terribly uncertain.

The perception of statistics is notoriously subjective.[3] In the 1980s I kept a folder of articles and stories labeled "Sick Docs," and my favorite was by a physician who believed he would die of his cancer. The five-year disease-free survival rate for his disease was 90%, and still he felt doomed. Then one day he realized that he "had decided, having been in the top 10 per cent of everything I did, that I would be the one in ten to die of this tumor."[4] After my daughter's diagnosis, the story wasn't charming anymore. I complained to my physician colleagues about breast cancer's relatively rotten statistics. A one-in-five chance of recurrence in five years—who knows beyond that— and, with microcalcifications all through the biopsied tissue, a second, equally strong chance—a new toss of the coin, unbiased by this occurrence—of a new cancer down the road. This was the best they could do?

It was the best they could do.

The best it can do is, at its best, what medicine does.

We make a great, even dangerous mistake about medicine when we assume it is a science in the realist Newtonian sense we learned in high school—even that it is, as Lewis Thomas described it, "the youngest science."[5] The words are noble and the aspirations praiseworthy, but assuming that medicine is a science leads to the expectation that physicians' knowledge is invariant, objective, and always replicable. Although biological research now provides the content for much of medicine, clinical knowing remains first of all the interpretation of what is happening with a particular patient and how it fits the available explanations. Such knowledge is still called an opinion; the skill used in arriving at that opinion is called judgment. In this, physicians resemble lawyers and judges, and medical rationality resembles jurisprudence. Both professions are engaged in practical reasoning, which, as Aristotle observes, is shared with practitioners of navigation and moral reasoning.[6] In these realms, knowing is particular, experiential, and conventionally agreed upon. Although areas of agreement may be large, even international and transcultural, physicians, lawyers, and moral reasoners nevertheless rely on skill and judgment that are taught and practiced, improved and clarified case by case.[7] Without a doubt, biology provides essential knowledge and promotes valuable technological advance, but medicine, like other practices— engineering, architecture, law—has a body of experiential, detail-driven wisdom. In this, clinicians are far more like naturalists or archeologists than like biochemists or physicists.

Meanwhile, the lump was undoubtedly there, and it was cancer.

She would die if it stayed.

Or would she?

Bernie Siegel, Andrew Weil, Caroline Myss, and Christian Science promise that mind and spirit can alter flesh, and I do in part believe it. But I wouldn't want to bet on it until I had to, not for my child, not on faith alone. The chances don't seem strong, especially if such faith is not already part of one's everyday practice. In life as in medicine, as I once heard a venerable surgeon say, "you have to proceed with the guidance of the knowledge you trust."

My folk belief and hers, as George Engel observed of our time, is Western scientific medicine.[8]

What should be done for a 28-year-old's breast cancer? It's widely held to be different from breast cancer in older women, but no one knows entirely how or why. Because there are very few cases in young women, research is difficult. Breast cancer for thirty-somethings is more frequent but still rare. There is occasionally a thirties bar, a mere sliver, on age-distribution graphs, but never one for the twenties. As a result, breast cancer in very young women is treated like other breast cancers. For the time being this makes sense. There is no reason (yet) not to, and besides, there is nothing else to do.

Surgery then. Lumpectomy and radiation? Or a modified radical mastectomy? Mastectomy with or without reconstruction? What sort of reconstruction after the never-quite-proven failure of silicone? Immediate reconstruction so as to minimize the sense of loss and mutilation? Or a delay so as to deal with the sense of loss and mutilation? Opinion varies.

Breast cancer long ago crossed the postmodern divide. Patients and their families have access to the statistical uncertainties of its treatment and prognosis, and because the therapeutic choices bear different weights in different lives, people with breast cancer undergo a sudden, staggering education aimed at enabling them to choose well. A friend who studies the discourse of breast cancer called with advice (" 'Discourse?' " my daughter e-mailed, "Great! 'Hello, I'm Fred, I'll be your tumor this year . . .' "): "You are entering a real thicket. Your heads will swim with minutiae you never wanted to know."

The possibility of a lumpectomy depends on the relative size of breast and tumor.[9] There are no clear choices beyond that. No rules, not many obvious bets. Just preferences and available clinical proficiency. Chemotherapy, indeed everything, depends on the stage of the disease, determined not only by tumor size but also by metastases and the presence of cancer cells in the lymph nodes beyond the breast in the armpit and upper arm. Positive nodes are the clue to a not-yet-identifiable metastasis: tumor cells have left the breast, ready to colonize. And the meaning of negative nodes? Researchers now think malignant cells have been leaving the tumor all along, but, if the nodes are negative, not in such numbers that they've taken hold—or not in an identifiable way.

The number of positive nodes counts a great deal. Once Halsted's radical mastectomy took all the nodes; the less severe, modified radical mastectomy leaves enough arm tissue for most people, after rehabilitation, to approximate normal movement. While lumpectomy with radiation to the tumor site proved to be as effective as the modified radical, the surgical excision of nodes went on impairing people who have had breast cancer. Negative or positive, out they came. Here, as in the rest of medicine, it has been difficult not to do everything that can possibly be done if it might prolong life. Clinical research regularly focuses on paring down a treatment either in its severity or in the descriptors caught in its predictive net so that (ideally) it can be given to fewer people in milder doses for a shorter time. Every possible node was once taken, then every node along the axillary vein, now only 10 in an *en bloc* resection, or increasingly, just one "sentinel node." Scaling back in this way took a long time. It was no doubt hard for a surgeon to leave a node that might be cancerous, but it is, after all, primarily a sign of disease and chemotherapy will eliminate it. And for many people, the axillary surgery has been the most disabling consequence of breast cancer: swollen arms, easily infected scratches. Even the removal of only 10 nodes means a permanent increase in the risk of infection from cuts and scratches and a prohibition against carrying any more than 15 pounds: a suitcase, a heavy briefcase, a couple of grocery sacks, a baby.

And microcalcifications? They used to be seen only in patients undergoing mastectomy, and when mammography first revealed that they exist in the absence of tumors, they were regarded as precursors of cancer and removed. Now they're left, watched, even in women under 35, whose dense breast tissue makes keeping track of them by mammogram uncertain. The meaning of the calcifications has changed. They are not "precancerous" now, but a risk factor: 20% of those who have them go on to develop breast cancer.

But she already has breast cancer!

The calcifications are still a predictor. The dice will be rolled again. They'll "watch it."

Some women, exhausted with waiting, losing bits of tissue to biopsy every year or two, chose prophylactic double mastectomy. But no mastectomy ever takes out all the breast tissue. Men have breast cancer.[10] People who have never had cancer find a lump on the chest wall; those who have had a mastectomy find recurrences in the scar.

As recently as the 1980s, if a tumor were small with no metastases and negative nodes, chemotherapy was thought to be unnecessary. But some people with small tumors had unexpected metastatic recurrences years later, and the cells from the new biopsy matched the old cancer. No one knows what the cancer cells were doing all that time. They were not "just circulating"; they were there somewhere, quiescent. No one knows what made them begin to grow again. Guidelines were changed in 1988. Now almost everyone with the most common kind of breast cancer, no matter how small, is treated with chemotherapy. It's not the tumor that's treated. By then it's gone. What is treated is the possibility that the cancer cells have left the tumor and migrated to the rest of the body. That's why it's called "adjuvant" treatment. It's a hedged bet: the chances of recurrence receive chemotherapy. The rest of the body is unfortunately in the way.

If consensus has been reached about who needs chemotherapy, there are nevertheless bewildering choices among chemotherapeutic agents and regimens. For my daughter, the decisions included timing. Should the chemotherapy come before radiation? After? Split around it? Four choices, and all that was known statistically about their consequences for longevity, fertility, and side effects (including subsequent, iatrogenic cancers) were laid out for her and her husband by a young oncologist who not only tolerated their need to understand what they were embarked upon but also encouraged it. Together they made a chart of the options: the standard, Cytoxan-Methotrexate-5-Flourouracil (CMF) every three weeks for six months, the newer, more caustic alternative, Adriamycin-Cytoxan (AC) every three weeks for three months, and two longer, experimental protocols, whose effects, under study, were not known. They added a fifth—no chemotherapy—for reference.

The thicket of nightmare possibilities, some of them contingent on others, puts breast cancer in the category of disease Lewis Thomas described as characterized by "halfway technology": high cost, elaborate and uncertain therapy, "at the same time highly sophisticated and profoundly primitive." For such diseases, Thomas observed, diagnosis and treatment involve highly trained personnel, special facilities and equipment, and enormous expense. The aim is not prevention or cure but "making up for the disease or postponing death."[11] The thickness of Susan Love's *Breast Book*, the lucid, authoritative guide to breast cancer and its treatment, is evidence of the mounds of information that a person may be called upon to reckon with. Although Love describes current areas of research and their goals, the book is inevitably out of date even as successive editions are printed.[12] Internet breast cancer groups help—and not only with the facts. They are especially recommended for younger people, who are better represented there than in face-to-face support groups. Besides, as my daughter observed, parodying the cartoon about the Internet, no one can see that you're bald.

The drive for information led her and her husband to their town library, where they read textbooks and got by heart the *New England Journal of Medicine's* recent summary article on breast cancer. By the time I got there before her surgery, they knew all the pathophysiology and had a good grasp of the pharmacology and sound instincts about the social customs. They had asked me to find in the medical library three studies the oncologist mentioned: a description of the chemotherapy regimen they chose, a study of birth defects in the children of cancer patients (insignificant for the drugs used to treat breast cancer), and the study that established that pregnancy does not accelerate tumor growth. I didn't go to the library for days. When I did, it was with a friend, then a resident, who coached me through the loss of what little facility I had had with on-line searches. The abstracts printed out were brutally plain: real lives aggregated into bare numbers. But they were no worse than a sentence glimpsed in a woman's magazine doing its Breast Cancer Month duty: only 65% of young women with breast cancer survive five years. When finally I went to the stacks, I read everything and found no comfort. Cancer cells have been studied by every characteristic they are now known to possess in a search for better predictors or a clue to new treatment. Estrogen and progesterone receptivity and DNA are just a start. High S-phase fractions, aneuploidy, HER-2/neu negativity, and estrogen-receptor negativity characterize breast cancer in young women. Bad as they are, they do not entirely add up: "Higher mortality in young women is not completely accounted for by the known prognostic factors." Studies continue, proliferate like the cells themselves. Bound together into volumes on library shelves, they are a massive reminder of the tentativeness of current scientific knowledge. Once breast cancer is understood right down to the bottom—etiology, diagnosis, therapy, and prognosis—it will take up a page and a half in a textbook. Still, the scientific journals were somehow reassuring. They're working on it, I told myself.

And they are. The nightmare thicket can be cleared. Much of it is, after all, the temporary uncertainty that comes from lack of knowledge at Thomas's "halfway" stage: what we know we don't know, answers to the questions even I might think of. This is not the uncertainty that finally must be confronted, however. What's even harder to think about is how uncertainly any of these numbers apply to one particular woman.

I walked, meditated, read Larry Dossey's clinical assessment of prayer.[13] I wrestled with the statistics: she's young and strong, she found it early, her doctors and nurses and technicians are very good, she had no nodes! But to no avail: 75% and 82% are numbers in a study of similar women, all of whom caught it early, all with stage I tumors, all receiving exactly the same therapy from physicians and nurses well-trained enough to undertake the studies. And "young" was not an advantage. I came to hate the walk from the hospital parking garage to my office. In that short block, my efforts at acceptance faded, and my hope of humbling myself—in a way that might alter fate—before the indifferent splendor of the universe dropped away. "Higher mortality in young women is not completely accounted for by the known prognostic factors" went round and round in my head. That is the science, such as it is, and in a medical school it demanded daily acknowledgment. Not that my physician-colleagues reminded me. They were far too kind.

I had gone over to the other side. I watched them shift, sometimes in the middle of a conversation, to regarding me as one of those others: a patient, a patient's mother. I battered them angrily with the facts of illness, vulnerability, medicine's imperfection.

Some of the imperfection is society's. While we often speak of medicine and society as if they were entirely distinct, encapsulated "influences" on one another, they are inseparably enmeshed. The United States took a long time to acknowledge breast cancer. It was a shameful secret until the 1970s, when Rose Kushner wrote *Why Me?*[14] and Betty Ford and Happy Rockefeller called press conferences in startling succession to talk about their diagnoses. They urged women to do self-exams and get mammograms but above all to regard breast cancer as a disease and not a failure of womanhood. Since then, the disease rate has risen from one in eleven in the early 1980s to almost one in eight. The increase feels like an epidemic. What the civil rights movement taught women about equal pay for equal work the gay community taught about research funding: politeness can be fatal. Until the infusion of funding in the early 1990s thanks to Congresswoman Patricia Schroeder and National Institutes of Health director Bernadine Healy, a sizable proportion of breast cancer research was conducted in Italy. The multicenter studies that established lumpectomy and radiation as an alternative to mastectomy were, in part, conducted there. The Cytoxan-Methotrexate-5-Florouracil regimen, standard chemotherapy for two decades, was developed there; so was Adriamycin, a poison named poetically, possessively, for the Adriatic. Meanwhile, in the United States, medicine was slow to give up the Halsted radical mastectomy, slow to adopt the breast-conserving lumpectomy, slow to devise new chemotherapy regimens, then slow to limit the number of nodes removed for staging, now slow to develop new tests. Breast cancer cells must shed *something* into the bloodstream, I'd challenge a colleague. Why isn't there a test?

The question of cause consumed me. What had gone wrong? A gene had mutated, cells had proliferated unchecked, but what had caused that? The possibilities—genetic inheritance, environmental and dietary carcinogens, stress—were numerous and slippery at best. My daughter's paternal aunt had died in her forties of ovarian cancer, but no genetic mutation thus far accounts for what is probably a coincidence. Our neighborhood in the 1980s had logged a case of breast cancer in every one of its ordinary-sized blocks of single-family houses, but so prevalent is breast cancer in the United States that this information is a better sign of a close-knit community than of an environmental cause. International studies have implicated the American diet. As an adult, my daughter ate relatively little fat, but her special treat as a child had been her baby sitter's own childhood favorite, stewed chicken necks and rice, until we learned the necks were the site of injections of diethylstilbestrol (DES), the growth hormone. She had spent seven years in New York City at increasingly stressful work, but she had no known occupational exposure. The cause that seemed most likely was iatrogenic: she had ingested radioactive iodine for Graves' disease two years before. The technician who administered it wore mask and gloves, and she herself was counseled not to touch anyone and to double-flush the toilet for three days afterward. Yet studies have not shown that this treatment increases the risk of breast cancer. Was it some combination of these things? Surely there was a cause that, if removed or reversed, could have kept her safe.

If the causes of breast cancer are inaccessible, what is known about en-couraging recovery, preventing recurrence? She reduced the meat and fat in her diet even further, ate more broccoli, cauliflower, and tofu, and developed an unlikely taste for soy milk. She went on exercising, learned biofeedback. Friends suggested meditation, visualization, prayer. Anxious for something, anything, that could be controlled, I imagined that the difference between the four in five who stayed well and the one in five who suffered a recurrence might be that the four had mothers who had faith: faith in God or, failing that, faith in medicine. What if some communicable maternal serenity in a mysterious way we don't yet understand strengthens the younger woman? Her mother *knows* she will be all right and so she is. In the days after the diagnosis, when the scans were still to be done and the positive node count was still weeks away, I spent a good while walking on the nearby beach. I had better sense than to ask Why me? Indeed the burning, terrible question was Why *not* me? Why my daughter? But whatever the question, the answer is eternally the same. I imagined it rumbling from beyond the horizon of Lake Michigan like a late summer squall: Why not? Only Job's answer was left me: to repent "in dust and ashes" of my question and its audacity. Still, at odd moments, doubled over, I found myself bargaining for her life, offering my body parts, my life, the hope of grandchildren, at last even her body parts. When I mentioned this odd new pastime, she wrote back, "As long as you're appealing to higher powers, don't compromise."

At the heart of the quest for certainty is a longing for control. Or, to look at it the other way around, we disguise the need for control as a need for knowledge. We don't have control. Nor are we likely to achieve it. We work hard to provide stability—the illusion of certainty—for our children. Parenthood is largely a matter of turning over this task to them, of preparing them for the gradual assumption of responsibility for their own lives. But we have no control. If we did, there would certainly be no breast cancer for 28-year-olds. But there might be no teenage driver's licenses, no camping expeditions across the country, no trips to China.

She had a lumpectomy, chemotherapy, radiation. The usual. Or, as Odetta keens through the first act finale of the Bill T. Jones/Arnie Zane dance suite, *Still/Here*: slash, poison, burn. I sat next to her as the Adriamycin snaked into her body. It is an antibiotic so toxically opposed to life that the nurse didn't let it drip along with the rest of the mix—saline, Cytoxan, Zofran, Decadron—but sat to push it slowly into the plastic tubing that ran into her arm. If a drop leaked it would destroy her flesh to the bone. I aligned myself with her so exactly that if by miracle it could have entered me instead it would have done it. It did not. A good friend, an internist whose daughter-in-law had just finished chemotherapy for breast cancer, wrote:

> Fear takes turns with rage and longing and magical thinking.
> Think of red Adriamycin as a magical potion.

E-mail turned it into a piece of a poem and I posted it where I could see it every day.

In the absence of magic, in the absence of certainty, I did other things. I requilted her childhood comforter, a project I had put off since it fell apart when she was 11 or 12 (it had been mine before that) and put off again from her departure for college through the first apartment of her own and then past her marriage. Until then. Once I sang to her as she lay inert with Ativan, the sledgehammer sedative she took for the violent nausea and vomiting. She was falling asleep, and I was trying to live out my premonitory dream in a way that didn't add up to dying. As cold weather closed in, I thought a lot about the myth of Demeter, a story that I had always believed belonged to her daughter Persephone: a young woman leaves home to see the world and assume her life as a sexual being; her mother gets upset. Now I saw it as Demeter's story after all. Wild with grief and rage at her child's abduction to the underworld, she decrees that there will be no spring until Persephone is returned from the clutches of Hades. I found Chicago's gray, cold weather strangely comforting.

Through the fall and winter, the *New England Journal of Medicine* regularly included ads for Kytril, the second of the new, "miracle" antiemetics. The first, Zofran, had changed the use of Adriamycin from a nearly intolerable treatment to (with Cytoxan) a real alternative to the old six-month-long warhorse, CMF, and here was an improvement. The Kytril ad was beautiful: two and a half pages, dense study results, and a picture of a golden, glorious sundial promising—what? Emergence into the sunlight? Sunny summer days?

I tore it out and pinned it above my desk as a promise that biomedical knowledge is advancing and that she'd be all right.

But she wasn't all right. She took the miraculous drug ($78 a pill) along with Ativan, the sedative of choice for detoxifying alcoholics, and the tranquilizer Compazene, but she had total-body nausea and vomiting that, while far short of the esophagus-rupturing damage Adriamycin is capable of, was still terrible. Despite adjustments in dosage, it worked even less well the second time, and her husband drove over icy rural Connecticut roads 15 minutes before the nearest pharmacy closed to buy Zofran, the "old" wonder drug, now reduced to $29 a pill. $740 spent on antiemetics in five hours. "What do people without insurance do!" my daughter exclaimed, knowing the answer. Zofran worked little better. With the third round of chemo, Compazene was replaced with a drug that unfocused her eyes and numbed her lower jaw. The vomiting went on.

Before the fourth round, I resolved to find some marijuana. Stephen Jay Gould wrote very little about his stomach cancer in the 1980s, but he described the experimental treatment he finally undertook, an early trial of Adriamycin. It made him so violently ill for so long that despite an adamant, lifelong resistance to any sacrifice of his rationality, he decided to smoke marijuana, and it enabled him to finish the treatment. I asked around and was promised some for my daughter. A generous ounce came stuffed into the spine of a recently published, respectable scholarly book by Lester Grinspoon and James B. Bakalar that argues for its medical use.[15] My friend wrapped the book in innocent homemade gift paper and tied it with a raffia bow.

Scientific research has cast doubt on marijuana as an antiemetic. Certainly the legally synthesized pill form called Marinol has not been shown to work. To be reliably therapeutic, pot must be smoked. The fantastic recipe for a hashish-laced confection in Alice B. Toklas's *Autobiography* and its mundane brownie variant deliver the dose too slowly and in an imprecisely controlled amount. Smoke, by contrast, works immediately and is easily adjusted. But it needs to be started before chemotherapy, and two days before I was to leave, four days before her chemotherapy, snow began to fall. Would the plan work? Would I get there in time? Physical certainty is no greater than certainty of clinical knowledge. In a year of failing airlines, I had a ticket that was still good. The plane would surely head in the right direction, almost certainly land. But, besides the snow, who knew what else might intervene: a traffic jam, a slip on the ice, a cold or flu I could pass on to my daughter in her immuno-compromised state. What in life is ever certain until it's pared down so small that it can be controlled? So small that we might not think it matters. That biomedical science can approximate that experimental control in a human body is a source of wonder. And gratitude, of course.

The wild card was a record-breaking blizzard. My flight was canceled. Airports throughout the East were closed for days. I felt sure I could drive there—less than a thousand miles. It was only snow, after all. But I had a saving suspicion that this was the operatic choice, that I was equally likely to end in a snow bank. I decided instead to trust that the snow would stop in time, that runways and roads would be cleared. While the snow fell, I carefully unwrapped the book, peered into the spine, and read every word, even the chapters on glaucoma. Two days later, almost as soon as the first runway was plowed, I made my way through Newark Airport. It was the morning of my daughter's appointment, and I had the goods on my middle-aged professorial person, along with 8 ounces of redolent candied ginger, a friend's recipe for gingersnaps (reputed to quell nausea), and a pound of pungent coffee beans for my son-in-law. The drug dogs, if they were interested, didn't stand a chance. Two lanes of the interstate were open, one in the right direction. While I made my way toward the hospital, the oncologist was explaining to them why she hadn't been given Marinol and that, if she used marijuana, she should omit the Ativan, not the miracle antiemetic. We wouldn't have known. The last difficulty was that my daughter, despite her inner-city public high school diploma and an excellent liberal arts education, had somehow never learned to smoke. But she had married a preacher's kid with briefly exercised but first-rate bong-making skills, and she let us coach her, never getting high, always choking, but not vomiting anymore either. "It's time for your pot," I heard myself saying once and added a quick, ironically maternal "dear."

It worked. "It keeps the nausea down where it belongs," she reported to an older sister three days later. "Almost controls it."

She has done well. She went on working, taking a few days off for surgery and each chemotherapy and a half day to be fitted for the radiation mold and marked for the lasers. Friends, so recently assembled for their wedding, came and called, sent flowers and lucky objects, wrote and e-mailed. Before chemotherapy, her husband cut her long hair twice—first to shoulder length, then just below her ears. Then she went with a friend to a hairdresser and came away with a half-inch buzz cut. The effect was dazzling. As planned, the family assembled at their new house for Thanksgiving. She asked for hats and was given a closetful. Her bald head, on a lifelong science fiction reader, was shockingly beautiful. She observed. She thought. She learned. She sent regular e-mail reports—"The Baldness Bulletin"—to family and her friends. She was cut but scarcely mutilated. She recovered from the poison.

The burning left small, ineradicable tattoos but no scars. April came. Her hair, beginning to grow back, approximated that dazzling buzz cut. Strangers asked her how she dared to do it, how she knew she'd look so great with such short hair. It had been an expensive hairstyle. Her energy, her creativity slowly returned. She and her husband were told to wait to have children, but they were young as parenthood is measured now. When the last treatment was done, the tulip bulbs they had sent me just before it all began were on the point of blooming. Spring.

Back at my writing table, computer on, notebooks open, I was afraid to read, really read, anything I had ever written about medicine's uncertainty. This book was mostly thought out, some of it written. I would easily have given it up in exchange for the certainty of her cure; I would deny everything I know about uncertainty if that could revoke its truth. But it also seemed that not to write the book would be a challenge to fate: a kind of hubris, still hoping for control. Instead, I have written it slowly, aware of the crisis of knowing that awaits those physicians who glimpse the disjunction between their idea of science and the medicine they practice. My hopes for medicine's science are challenged by what I know about medicine's practice. Research will increase our knowledge of breast cancer, I have no doubt. My daughter donated an aliquot—they still use that old-fashioned word—of blood to a study of the disease in very young women. We will know more: we already know more in the time since she made her choices. Will we know more in her lifetime? In time to save her if her cancer recurs? There's the question.

No one knows.

The practice of medicine, even in the era of postmodern cultural studies, is irreducibly material, real. The body is there: alive, beyond construction or representation, although unknown without those human acts. Bodies bear our identity, are our selves; they are socially constructed but not out of nothing. Bodies are language, mute appeal for recognition, for attention and care. Knowledge may be contingent, and existence may be too, but bodies are given: needy, playful, pleasurable, healthy, ill. They are interpreted, treated, sometimes cured. In its response to a suffering human being, medicine works upon the body, attends the person, at its best buoys the spirit. There is always the hope of going on, of knowing more.

Knowing in medicine, a science of individuals, is a two way, bidirectional matter. What can be drawn from the individual experience? Can it be generalized? Abstraction from the particular case is always a problem in medicine. What did her sudden loss of energy 10 days after the first chemotherapy mean? Why did her hands bruise easily for a long time afterward? The usefulness of established abstractions is a puzzle too: how does general, scientific knowledge apply to her particular case? Why did marijuana, which has been declared ineffective, stop her nausea when two well-studied antiemetics with Food and Drug Administration (FDA) approval did not? Regular scans determined that Adriamycin didn't damage her heart. But what about other damage? The radiation that cures cancer causes it too. The statistical chances of developing leukemia after exposure are known rad by rad. What are her chances? How do they compare to those of an eastern European under Chernobyl rainfall?

When we know more, will we have control? And for everyone? There will always be mistakes, delays, and, worst, the persistent assumption that a lump in a 28-year-old's breast—or a man's—is surely nothing to worry about. Tumors will be more and less accessible; breasts will vary in size and density. The red Adriamycin now and then will leak. Women will vary in their willingness to be tested and, so long as the cost of tests stays elevated to amortize the oversupply of mammogram machines, in their ability to pay for it. Judgment calls on breast signs are still unstudied. Radiologists, for example, will differ in the interpretation of scattered calcifications: some will be "insufficiently suspicious"; some will cross a line and be biopsied. What constellation of bright specks becomes sufficiently suspicious? Where, what is that line? For which physician? With regard to which women?

Biomedicine will know much more: about the etiology, the genetics, the immunology, about timely and nonmutilating diagnosis, effective treatment, cultural variants in diagnosis and treatment, and the psychosomatic components of the disease. Medicine will even learn more about the sensitivity and specificity of radiologists' interpretations. We may adopt a therapeutic practice from another country or discover for ourselves a prophylactic herb—or, who knows, go on eating broccoli to good effect. Someone may demonstrate, as David Spiegel was believed to have done for support groups, that meditation or prayer increase life expectancy for the seriously ill.[16] Society may even learn to celebrate, as Audré Lorde challenges us to do, the one-breasted woman.[17]

All we learn will work better than what we know now. But it will never be certain knowledge. Medicine will never know everything for every case, and the knowledge physicians have will not always translate into effective action. It won't be control—nor even, in and of itself, power. I once teased a not-quite-40-year-old friend who had had a bone marrow transplant for breast cancer for worrying that her hands were a little stiff in the morning: did she think coming through all those deadly chemicals, all that suffering, would keep her from getting older? Not aging was the *other* possibility, the fate she had so far avoided. The rest of life's chances remained.

What acceptance of uncertainty I managed that year I learned from the younger generation. Ten days after the diagnosis, my daughter reported an odd happiness: "At first I felt like it didn't matter what happened to me because all of a sudden I had this fatal disease. Maybe I should learn to rock climb because I wouldn't be so scared to die. After all, I'm going to anyway, perhaps sooner than expected. That was sort of interesting. Now I feel more like I should take Very Good Care of Myself—not because I feel fragile or accident prone, but because now that it looks like I'll get through all this pretty well, it would be a shame to get hit by a bus covered with Snapple ads on Third Avenue."

Just before the surgery, well before the physical toll began but with the therapeutic course more or less mapped out, her husband said, "The odds just seem to sharpen life's chances. They're bearable." He paused. "I'm thinking hard about the Quaker advice to be thankful in all things."

Beyond the search for accurate predictors, uncertainty remains—to say nothing of blizzards and the bus tearing past on Third Avenue.

For now, breast cancer is forever. Five-year disease-free survival is just that. There is no cure. I follow the biological research, now wonderfully energized by an infusion of funding. I admire the work of Hollis Siegler, who has made the postmastectomy body the theme of her art, and of Matuschka, who bared her scarred chest on the cover of the *New York Times Magazine* and dared us to look away.[18] The genes BRCA-1 and BRCA-2 have been located and pathogenic mutations identified. Research has established that a normal, unmutated BRCA gene produces a protein that reduces tumors in mice. What all this means for my daughter I can scarcely bear to think. More is known now, but medicine is not simply these scientific discoveries. Further discoveries will not grant certainty to a particular patient. Far from being an objective observer of medicine, for a long time I alternately raged at it and wanted to give up all I know in exchange for simple trust.

She has had the best medical care there is. But the best treatment for breast cancer is still primitive, barbaric, and uncertain. Some day the women who have survived it will regale their granddaughters with accounts of the weird things done back at the turn of the millennium. How can I have faith in those treatments? Someone whose child is in peril and who knows too much about medicine is challenged by a version of the awful awareness that physicians somehow manage to overcome or ignore. It is the irony of medicine. Medicine is not a science; physicians must act. They must do the best they can, even when it is inadequate, even when they don't know all there is to know, even when there is nothing to do. So must we all.

CHAPTER TWO

⌒⌒

The Misdescription of Medicine

To say that all human thinking is essentially of two kinds—
reasoning on the one hand, and narrative, descriptive,
contemplative thinking on the other—is to say only
what every reader's experience will corroborate.

—WILLIAM JAMES

IF MEDICINE IS not a science, what is it?

Once in the mid-1980s, at a clinical research conference I attended every week, I observed aloud that medicine has the methodology, the rationality, of the social sciences. I meant to make a useable point about my colleagues' approach to some matter at hand, but it was quickly brushed aside as the mistake of a clueless outsider. Lucky thing. I was near the beginning of three years of clinical observation. Although I was a faculty member in the medical school, they regarded me (quite rightly) as a learner. Only the National Science Foundation grant funding my research guaranteed that I was worth setting straight. I did not know then that the eminent medical historian Henry Sigerest, himself a physician, had made the same observation. "Medicine," he said, "is not so much a natural as a social science."[1] I've wondered since whether it would have made much difference if I had been able to cite Sigerest on the spot. My colleagues were clinical researchers concerned with establishing a solid academic reputation for what was then a new whole-patient, primary care specialty, general internal medicine. Although they undoubtedly revered the great men of medicine, I suspect they would have dismissed someone who had written in the 1940s and 1950s, before the advent of truly advanced, technologically sophisticated medicine.

Twenty years after my colleagues' charitable dismissal, the description of medicine as a social science still has little appeal. Within the profession and in society at large, the everyday understanding of physicians' work is still lodged in descriptions that are crude, incomplete, and unreflective. Medicine is described as a science, and if that description is qualified, usually on ritual occasions, it is with the assertion that it is also an art.[2] Commencement speakers are fond of invoking the two in quick succession without much definition of either term. "Medicine is a science," graduating physicians are reminded, "but it is an art as well." Or the duality is posed the other way around. "Medicine is an art," the speaker will say, adding soon after, "but above all, of course, it is a science." These descriptions are not so much wrong as ill-defined and shallow. They are a reminder that medicine, site of modern miracles, is poorly defined and poorly described by those who nevertheless practice it quite well.

Medicine as a Science and an Art?

The paradox of "art" and "science" in descriptions of medicine points to a tension in medicine itself. Indeed, that tension is undoubtedly what commencement speakers are attempting to capture and, sometimes, celebrate. Good medicine is a rational practice based on a scientific education and sound clinical experience. It is neither an art nor a science. Or, it seems, if it is one of them, it must also be the other.

The terms themselves are slippery and almost entirely unexamined.[3] Along with "wisdom," "intuition," and "talent," Donald Schön lists "artistry" as one of the terms typically used as a "junk category" to describe what cannot be "assimilate[d] to the dominant model of professional knowledge."[4] On ritual occasions, "the art of medicine" may refer to behavioral attributes such as bedside manner or the display of professional etiquette. Or it may designate moral values or virtues manifested in demeanor or habits of communication. It can be any or all of those aspects of physicianhood that seemed squishy and inessential during medical school. All are recognizably different from the knowledge of biology. More usefully, "art" stands for the relatively subjective skills of physical diagnosis or, more precisely, for tacit knowledge, the hunches that experienced physicians have without quite knowing how. Described as intuition (now that this once gender-laden word is allowed) essential to good practice, those "gut feelings" are a sort of know how: as nonscience, this must be art.

The common understanding of "science" in medicine is equally odd. Whether referring to biomedicine, to technology, or to the rational procedures of clinical work, the word promises the unambiguous regularities of Newtonian physics. Journalists and schoolteachers, as well as random people in the street, assume that science is the replicable, invariant, universalizable description of material reality. "Science" denotes the laws by which the physical world works, laws so regular that particular details can be invariably deduced from them. Even people who have learned from studies in the history or philosophy or sociology of science that it is far more complicated default to this positivist view, just as every post-Copernican speaks of the sun "coming up" in the morning and "going down" at the end of the day. With medicine, the intellectual anachronism seems justified by the years physicians spend studying human biology: anatomy, histology, physiology, microbiology and virology, pathology, pharmacology, and, more recently, molecular biology. But biology is more complex and variable than the physical sciences that medicine idealizes, and human biology is even more multilevel than that.[5] "Science," especially in its limited, old-fashioned physics-based sense, is neither an adequate description of what physicians do nor a good characterization of how they think. Some physicians are engaged in bench research, of course, and in their labs they are scientists. They conduct biological experiments or design Phase I clinical trials, and, like their scientist-colleagues with Ph.D.s, these physician-experimenters are rightly concerned with replicability and generalizability. As scientists, the individual case is of necessity not their first concern.

Medicine is different. When physicians who conduct research turn to their clinical duties, they are no longer scientists but clinicians: physicians who take care of patients. Even if every one of a physician's patients is enrolled in an experimental protocol, the ethics of medicine decrees that with regard to those patients the physician is first and foremost a physician and not a research scientist. The language reflects the distinction: "Medical science" is what goes on in laboratories and on computers, while "scientific medicine" means the well-informed care of patients. For the practitioner, "medicine" remains the substantive; "scientific" is its modifier. George Bernard Shaw's *Doctors' Dilemma* (1906) and Sinclair Lewis's *Arrowsmith* (1925) both turn upon a physician's temptation to abandon this fundamental difference. So does the disgrace of the Tuskegee syphilis study. In Lewis's novel, a clash between science and medicine fuels the crisis for its hero, who has adopted both callings. In the midst of a bubonic plague epidemic on a Caribbean island, Martin Arrowsmith abandons his investigation of a promising new therapy and allows desperate people in his control group to receive the test vaccine. He cannot be sure he is saving lives, but he endangers his scientific career to respond to people who come to him for help. The Tuskegee study went the other way. Patients—or, rather, the men who were its subjects—were denied the newly discovered penicillin so as not to interrupt a study of the natural course of untreated syphilis. It stands as a reminder of the inescapable, necessary difference between science and medicine.

The passage of time will not alter this difference. Medicine is not a science, not in the positivist sense that is customarily meant. While diagnosis and treatment have become intensely science-using activities, those activities are not in and of themselves science.[6] Nor does the unavoidably experimental nature of clinical practice qualify medicine as a science. It is true that no treatment prescribed to an individual patient is ever entirely certain in its effect, but that is clinical, not scientific, experimentation, with variables that are beyond control. Physicians start from the demands of the patient's condition and not from the demand for generalizable knowledge, and their goal is just as particular: to treat the patient's illness, not to test the therapy. They cannot begin by reasoning from the general rule to the particular case because biological laws are too abstract and imprecise to be applied uniformly to every patient. Instead they must reason from the particular to the general and then (for confirmation) back again. They start with the details of the present illness—is the pain sharp or dull? what makes it better?—all the while fitting the answers into a complex and general taxonomy of paradigm cases of disease. Because understanding an individual instance of illness requires an inquiry into its circumstances, diagnosis is an interpretive negotiation of the particular signs and symptoms and their development over time. The goal is their narrative coherence in a diagnosis that accounts for all the evidence. Medicine, if it is a science, is that oxymoron, a science of individuals, which Aristotle in the *Metaphysics* declared was an impossibility.[7]

The science-art duality is surely inspired by a sense of this oddity. It signals that medicine is recognizably different from science pure and simple. Commencement speakers stop there, but the duality—the paradox—is central to understanding the nature of medicine. It participates in the "binary economy" that Caroline Jones and Peter Galison identify as a conventional image in Western culture, one that animated C. P. Snow's mid-twentieth-century two-cultures debate. "Like all binaries," Jones and Galison say, "art and science [need] to be yoked together (yet held apart) in order to accrue the strengths of their polar positions: soft versus hard, intuitive versus analytical, inductive versus deductive, visual versus logical." The interesting questions, as they go on to explore, arise from the intersection of the two.[8] And so it is in medicine, where the impossibility of being at once a science and an art cries out for explication. Failing to receive that attention—for those who use the duality sometimes elaborate but never examine it—the image survives, just barely viable, as cliché. Medicine is left facilely described and, on the evidence, poorly understood.

The extent of the effect this misrepresentation of medicine has on its practice is difficult to know, but the science-art paradox has one consequence that is probably unintended by the honored medical elders who invoke it. It creates distinct and difficult-to-reconcile aspects of medicine—unequal ones at that—and suggests that they function as alternatives. Those who speak of the art and science of medicine do not suggest that the two exist on a continuum: the more art, the less science, and vice versa. Instead, it is as if they were one of those goblet-or-profiles illusions: impossible to see at the same time, incommensurable, important in distinct and quite dissimilar situations. This irreconcilable split is echoed in the heat of medical faculty battles, when those advocating that scarce curriculum time be given to the humanities or social sciences are likely to be challenged with the mutually excluding question: Would you rather have a physician who is skilled or one that will hold your hand? It is a false choice, as most commencement speakers would agree, but how is the question to be answered when it cannot be literally true that an activity is at once an art and a science?

The Exercise of Clinical Judgment

What is neglected by the science-art duality is medicine's character as a practice. It is far more than a body of scientific knowledge and a collection of well-practiced skills, although both are essential. It is the conjunction of the two: the rational, clinically experienced, and scientifically informed care of sick people. Its essential virtue is clinical judgment, the practical reasoning or phronesis that enables physicians to fit their knowledge and experience to the circumstances of each patient.[9] Details of human biology and countless bits of technological information are called from memory, along with their own experiences and those reported by others, and the whole is focused by (and on) the details of a particular patient's illness.

Aristotle describes phronesis in the *Nicomachean Ethics* as the intellectual capacity or virtue that belongs to practical endeavors rather than to science.[10] Although twenty-first-century beneficiaries of science are not much used to thinking of different kinds of rationality, phronesis or practical reasoning is nevertheless a valuable, even a familiar concept. As an interpretive, making-sense-of-things way of knowing, practical rationality takes account of context, unpredicted but potentially significant variables, and, especially, the process of change over time. Yet in most accounts of medicine, phronesis or clinical judgment is set aside in favor of the conventional binary split between knowledge of the hard, reliable stuff and the mushy but unavoidable ineffabilities. Still, there it is, at the intersection of scientific knowing and craft-skill: clinical judgment, the goal of medical education and the pride of expert physicians.

Why is clinical judgment not celebrated? These days, physicians may no longer see a comparison of clinical medicine with social science or skepticism about its claims to be a science as attacks on their profession, but those views are still regarded as the peculiar opinions of a nonphysician. A celebration of clinical judgment is likely to be seen as ignorance or the dismissal of science, a disregard for evidence, if not an outright return to the days of bleeding and leeches. For within the profession, medicine's shortcomings as a science are held to be local or temporary. Many of them are. Individual physicians may lack knowledge, especially early in their careers, and a few hours in the library or a few years of practice will supply the deficit. For the profession as a whole, there remain clinical puzzles to be solved and scientific advances to be made. But the assumption that everything about disease and injury in individual patients eventually will be known, quantified, and predicted is an unwarranted leap. Evidence-based medicine promises to refine knowledge and its application but not to supply complete information for every patient in each phase of any condition. Yet when doubt about the possibility of the ultimate perfection of knowledge enters the physician's mind, it is more likely to be prompted by the unyielding puzzle of a patient with a fever of unknown origin or an optimistic prediction that artificial intelligence (AI) will someday substitute for expert clinical practice than by the recollection of an undergraduate course in the philosophy of science.

Physicians are right about artificial intelligence, at least as we presently conceive of it.[11] If medicine were a science in the old-fashioned positivist sense, its laws could be programmed, and diagnosis could be determined and choice of treatment decided entirely by computer. There would be no need for physicians.[12] But even if computer programs, like textbook descriptions or the protocols given to emergency medical technicians, worked most of the time, they would still be an inadequate substitute for clinical attention. The need for human contact by both parties to the patient-physician encounter goes well beyond the patient's need for reassurance and support. Clinicians need to examine the patient for themselves. Not even acknowledged experts are comfortable venturing a diagnosis without firsthand knowledge. What experienced clinicians possess, with or without information gleaned from the latest journal article, is an immense and well-sorted catalogue of clinical cases and the clinical judgment to know how to use it, and that store of knowledge is activated by seeing, touching, and questioning the patient.

Such knowledge is varied and extensive enough so that the bottom-up rules of practice or maxims that the cases collectively embody are hedged and qualified, layered in memory with skepticism about their applicability to any particular patient. Solid attempts have been made in computer science to codify clinical expertise, but expert systems in medicine perform only at the level of a good intermediate practitioner and are no match for the expert. Patricia Benner's study of clinical expertise suggests the reason for this. The acquisition of clinical skill is a process that goes beyond mastery of rules, she claims, to a stage where the rules are no longer recalled; each case is comprehended wholistically.[13] The inability of clinical experts to identify general rules that guide them once prompted Edward Feigenbaum, an originator of artificial intelligence, to remark of physicians, "At this point, knowledge threatens to become ten thousand special cases." Hubert Dreyfus and Stuart Dreyfus—the former a philosopher who has long criticized AI as insufficiently contextual, the latter an applied mathematician whose work on expertise Benner uses—agree. They maintain that experts reason not by methodical inference but "holographically," and therefore Feigenbaum's frustration is an accurate description of the difficulties faced by those who would model clinical expertise.[14]

Not that computerized expert systems are not useful. Clinicians, when colleagues ask, are willing to suggest possible diagnoses based on an account of a case, and a good computer program can serve the same purpose. Still, as a replacement for the clinical encounter from start to finish, a clinical reasoning machine remains improbable. Either it would be a parodic sketch of the patient-physician encounter or it would cheat by requiring a clinician to supply the data, interpreting it in the process. To work well in medicine, AI needs just those laws that could establish medicine as a science, and in medicine such laws, like similar abstractions in history, economics, or political science, are increasingly useless in a practical sense the more general they become. Conversely, the more reliable they are, the less generalizably law-like they become and the fewer patients to whom they will apply. Physicians readily grasp this difficulty. It replicates the trade-off between sensitivity and specificity they are familiar with in diagnostic testing, a trade-off the rest of us know best from airport scanners or car alarms. Their understanding of the impossibility of achieving covering laws in medicine undergirds many of the attacks on evidence-based medicine or (more accurately placed) on its use by third-party payers. Yet physicians go on accepting descriptions of medicine as a science. They dismiss doubts about its scientific status by appealing to the probability calculations of epidemiology as a surrogate, approximate certainty;[15] or they optimistically predict that medicine's nonscientific subjectivity is a temporary flaw, an irrationality that will disappear when the last biological puzzle has been solved.

If clinical medicine is not an invariant and wholly predictive science now that it has become highly scientific and supremely technological, then further advances in science and technology are not likely to make it one. This is in part because scientific reasoning of the positivist, objective, replicable sort has only a small place in clinical practice. As patients, we know this. We don't look for a scientist when we are sick, not unless we are dying without recourse and there is news of some long-shot, potential remedy taking shape in the laboratory. People dying of cancer in the spring of 1998 were willing to take angiostatin—capable of stopping the blood supply to tumors in mice—straight from the bench scientist's vials. Supplying the substance to sick people would not have been medical treatment. At best, it would have been a clinical experiment, an unauthorized, premature Phase I trial, the kind that establishes drug toxicity in human beings (relevant animal research having been successfully completed) without any expectation of benefit to the experimental subject. That is scarcely what is meant by—or hoped for from— medicine. Physicians are expected to care for their patients and treat them more comprehensively. They must understand human biology, investigate the patient's condition attentively, reach a diagnosis, understand the clinical research and its relevance to the particular individual who is the patient, and then weigh the benefits and burdens of therapeutic choices and adjust the treatment as events unfold. Such a practice is certainly rational, but it is not (especially by medicine's own positivist definition) science.

Medicine, then, is a learned, rational, science-using practice that describes itself as a science even though physicians have the good sense not to practice that way.[16] This complexity may be close to what those who invoke the science-art duality are trying to express. After four years of instilling in their students both the habits of clinical reasoning and the belief that what they are doing is a science, on graduation day, medicine's elders publicly acknowledge that, although science remains the "gold standard," it is an inadequate description of all they hope new graduates have learned. As they leave for residencies, new physicians must know the science, of course, and also grasp what is meant by the art. What goes unspoken is that, because medicine is a practice in which rules must be applied interpretively, they must learn to negotiate the intersection of the two. They need to have developed the beginnings of good clinical judgment, sound practical reasoning. Yet the science-art duality persists long after graduation day, and the custom of splitting medicine into two parts shortchanges both the still neglected phenomenon of clinical reasoning and the difficult practical education in which new physicians are still immersed.

The Complexity of Clinical Rationality

Given the radical uncertainty of clinical medicine as a science-using practice that must diagnose and treat illnesses one by one, the complex reasoning physicians use requires a richer concept of rationality than a spare, physics-based, positivist account of scientific knowing. Kirsti Malterud argues that traditional medical epistemology is an inadequate representation of medical knowledge because "the human interaction and interpretation which constitutes a considerable element of clinical practice cannot be investigated from that epistemic position."[17] In view of this misrepresentation of clinical knowing, Eric Cassell has called instead for a bottom-up, experience-based theory of medicine:

> Knowledge . . . whether of medical science or the art of medicine, does not take care of sick persons or relieve their suffering; clinicians do in whom these kinds of knowledge are integrated. . . . [M]edicine needs a systematic and disciplined approach to the knowledge that arises from the clinician's experience rather than artificial divisions of medical knowledge into science and art.[18]

Such experienced knowing is clinical judgment, the exercise of practical reasoning in the care of patients. It is essential to medicine and its characteristic tasks: first (as Edmund Pellegrino enumerates them) to diagnose the patient, second, to consider the possible therapies, and finally to decide what is best to do in this particular circumstance.[19] By their nature, these are complex and potentially uncertain tasks, no matter how advanced the science that informs them, and the phronesis or clinical judgment they require is the essential virtue of the good physician. It is the goal toward which clinical education and the practice of medicine strive.

Complexity and uncertainty are built into the physician's effort to understand the particular in light of general rules. If physicians could be scientists, they surely would be. The obstacle they encounter is the radical uncertainty of clinical practice: not just the incompleteness of medical knowledge but, more important, the imprecision of the application of even the most solid-seeming fact to a particular patient. The development of epidemiology and strategies for its use with individual patients such as clinimetrics, clinical epidemiology, medical decision-making, and evidence-based medicine (EBM) have reduced this uncertainty and vastly improved patient care. Following on decades of clinical research, the Cochrane Collaboration's evaluation and reconciliation of the results of disparate, apparently incommensurable studies has encouraged the sense that by using the strategies of EBM, invariant precision—real certainty—in dealing with human illness may be just around the corner.[20] Although EBM has never claimed that, its impossibility is no reason not to work toward greater reliability in diagnosis, treatment, and prognosis. But, like the distance between Achilles and the tortoise, the gap between invariant, reliable, universalizable laws and the variable manifestations of illness in a particular patient remains. That is the nature of a science of individuals. We want it to be otherwise, especially when those we love or we ourselves are ill. But despite medicine's miracles—and they are legion—clinical knowing is not certain, nor will it ever be.

Scientific advance will not change this. In that ideal future when the pathophysiology of disease is thoroughly known and the epidemiology of every malady established, and both are at the fingertips of the experienced practitioner, medicine will remain a practice. Diagnosis, prognosis, and treatment of illness will go on requiring interpretation, the hallmark of clinical judgment. Physicians will still be educated and esteemed for the case-based practical reasoning that is situated, open to detail, flexible, and reinterpretable, because their task will continue to be the discovery of what is going on with each particular patient. Even with the last molecular function understood, the genome fully explicated, and cancer curable, the care of sick people will not be an unmediated "application" of science. People vary; diseases manifest themselves in varying ways. The individual patient will still require clinical scrutiny, clinical interpretation. The history will be taken, the body examined for signs, tests performed, and the medical case constructed. Patients will go on presenting demographically improbable symptoms of diseases; some will require toxic therapy, and sometimes treatment will come too late. Tests will have to be balanced between their sensitivity to marginal cases and the specificity with which they can identify disease. Therapies of choice will be second choice for some patients and will never cure quite everyone. The attentive focus on the particular patient that is the clinician's moral obligation will continue to compel the exercise of practical reason.

Because the practice of medicine requires the recollection and representation of subjective experience, physicians will go on investigating each clinical case: reconstructing to the best of their ability events of body, mind, family, and environment. For this task scientific knowledge is necessary and logic essential, even though the task itself is narrative and interpretive. Clinicians must grasp and make sense of events occurring over time even as they recognize the inherent uncertainty of this quasi-causal, retrospective rational strategy. Piecing together the evidence of the patient's symptoms, physical signs, and test results to create a recognizable pattern or plot is a complex and imprecise exercise. It is subject to all the frailty of historical reconstruction, but it remains the best—the logical, rational best—that clinical reasoners can do. It is not science, not in any positivist sense, nor is it art.

The Misrepresentation of Clinical Rationality

Why does medicine collude in the misrepresentation of its rationality? One obvious explanation is that medicine's status in society depends in large part on the scientific character of much of its information. To claim to be a scientist in our culture is to stake out authority and power. But physicians suffer the ill effects of this hubris: as patients and as citizens, we expect them to be far more certain than either their practice or the biology on which it is based can warrant, and, for many reasons, they are likely to take these expectations for their own. Malpractice suits that arise more from anger over misplaced expectations and perceived neglect than from genuine mistakes are the result.[21] As for power, it arises more strongly from human need in time of illness than from science. A widespread appreciation of clinical judgment would provide physicians a human and fallible but still trustworthy authority.

A more interesting, less obvious reason for describing medicine as a science is a practical requirement of clinical medicine, its need for certainty when taking action on behalf of another human being. Hans-Georg Gadamer describes such a need (though not the accompanying claim to science) as characteristic of all practice. "Practice requires knowledge," he writes, "which means that it is obliged to treat the knowledge available at the time as complete and certain."[22] Certainly one of medicine's chief strategies for minimizing the inescapable uncertainty of its practice is to regard—though always with skepticism—the best available information as real, dependable, and absolute, and these qualities are held to be characteristic of science. This practical strategy makes sense of an odd phenomenon: physicians' lack of interest in the late twentieth-century debate about the status of scientific knowledge or its representation of reality. Despite stereotypes about premedical students, many physicians have had a good liberal education, and all of them have met up with the assumption-rattling puzzle of quantum mechanics in the physics courses required for medical school admission. With their white coats off, they are likely to know as much about the history and philosophy of science as other college graduates. They nevertheless seem to need the honorific label "science" as a warrant for their clinical acts. Medical students who as undergraduates were immersed in philosophy or anthropology or cultural studies are no more likely to resist the science claim (with or without the art hedge) than those who majored in biomechanical engineering or economics. Once in practice, many physicians well educated in the biological sciences and keenly aware of the ineradicable uncertainty of their work still refer to medicine as a science—and without an apparent shred of epistemological doubt. It is as if, having embarked on a perilously uncertain practice, characterized by ungeneralizable rules and exceptions to those rules that proliferate like epicycles of the planets in Ptolemaic cosmology, they must cling for intellectual justification—beyond the need for social and interpersonal power—to the shards of a historical but by now metaphoric and inapplicable certainty.

Science is regarded as the "gold standard" of clinical medicine precisely because it promises reliability, replicability, objectivity—in short, what certainty is available in an uncertain practice. The metaphor of the gold standard, so widely used as an image of best practice and scientific certainty, is ironically apt—and just as unexamined as the science claim. Gold no longer backs any major world currency. It has gone the way of positivist science. Like science and the popular conception of rationality it stands for, gold is still available for the invocation of value, but it was long ago relativized, rendered conditional, and understood as in part the product of its social use.

One other reason for medicine's misdescription is an ethical one. Physicians argue that the belief that medicine is a science is essential to medical education. Clinical knowledge, although evolving, is at any given moment fixed and certain, and as teachers they want to foster in their students and residents a nearly obsessive attention to detail, a drive to know all that can be known, and a dedication to the best possible care for each patient. These are the marks of the good clinician. It might seem outrageous to ask them simultaneously to acknowledge clinical medicine's irreducible uncertainty—although, as I will show, covertly they manage to do exactly that at every clinical turn. Patients are resistant too. Do we want physicians to tell us as they enter the examination room that their knowledge is incomplete, its application to our case will be imprecise, and its usefulness uncertain? Not unless our complaint is very minor we don't. We want to think of them as powerful, dedicated, perfect figures. This rigid expectation carries over into the smallest details of education and practice. Work shifts for physicians and 80-hour weeks for residents have been resisted because they might limit their all-out dedication to patients. And patients, even when they know the assertion is necessarily suspect, still want to go on hearing "We've done everything possible." Few clinicians—or patients—have imagined changing this *folie a deux.*[23]

Is it possible to educate good physicians while recognizing that science is a tool rather than the soul of medicine? I believe it is, especially if that education were framed formally, as it now is tacitly, as a moral education, a long and scrupulous preparation to act wisely for the good of their patients in an uncertain field of knowledge.[24] A first step would be to scrap the unexamined description of clinical medicine as both a science and an art. The duality ignores all that medicine shares with moral reasoning and reinforces the contemporary tendency to split ethics from medicine. Moral knowing is the essence of clinical method, inextricably bound up with the care of the patient. In medicine, morality and clinical practice require phronesis, the practical rationality that characterizes both a reliable moral agent and a good physician.

Accounts of clinical medicine should celebrate clinical judgment and not the idea of science that physicians borrow from Newtonian physics. Nor should they appeal to a vaguely defined "art" to modify or enrich that outmoded idea of science. Clinical medicine is best described, instead, as a practice. Accounts of physicians' work, especially celebratory ones, should emphasize the exercise of clinical reasoning or phronesis, the deployment of clinical judgment on behalf of the patient. In equipping physicians to perform that essential task, medical education is necessarily a moral education, for it is training to choose what is best to do in the world of action. Its goal is the cultivation of phronesis, the practical reason essential to clinical judgment. The practice of medicine requires knowledge of human biology, a store of clinical experience, good diagnostic and therapeutic skills, and a familiarity with the vagaries of the human condition. Their intersection in the care of patients—the practice that makes physicians who and what they are—is neither a science nor an art. It is a distinctive practical endeavor whose particular way of knowing—its phronesiology—qualifies it to be that impossible thing, a science of individuals.

CHAPTER THREE

⌒⌒

Clinical Judgment and the
Interpretation of the Case

"Well, you know, Standish, every dose you take is
an experiment, you know—an experiment . . ."

—GEORGE ELIOT

IN A HAND-WRITTEN chart my daughter, her husband, and the oncologist laid
out her treatment options and what was known about the side effects of each.
But about her particular experience or her fate the chart had nothing to say.
Clinical medicine could diagnose her breast cancer and provide information
about its treatment, even offer a choice among several possibilities, but it could
not tell what had caused her tumor or say whether she would be among those
who survive. Indeed, she had her choice of treatments precisely because so
much was uncertain and because, in the judgment of her physicians, none of
them had a better clinical outcome than another.

The human need for certainty obscures the circumstantial nature of clinical medicine. Patients and physicians alike want medicine to be more certain
than it is, and as a result, few of either group are motivated to understand
how physicians acquire and use their knowledge.[1] An account of clinical
judgment—the practical reasoning necessitated by the absence of certainty—
is central to that effort. To some, the days of clinical judgment are numbered.
For them, evidence-based medicine (EBM) and its emphasis on the results
of clinical research promise to clarify and rationalize clinical reasoning to the
point of certainty, and expose clinical judgment as a disguise for old-fashioned
appeals to custom and authority. And while it is true that EBM's statistical

sophistication enables physicians to apply research with more subtlety and precision to an individual patient, it will not turn medicine into a science. Neither EBM's method nor the information it yields can do the work of clinical thinking alone. The answers it provides are useless without a clearly asked clinical question, and that is the province of clinical judgment.[2] The understanding of a patient's condition needed to formulate that question requires clinical experience, a store of well-sorted preliminary information, careful, even skeptical observation, a nuanced recognition of variation and anomaly, and the ability to put all this together. Any description of the discipline of medicine or the clinical judgment essential to its practice must take into account the convergence of these formative elements and the clinician's complex though rapid, habitual, and usually unnoticed negotiation among them.[3]

To understand the nature of clinical judgment, Aristotle's account of practical reasoning is a useful place to start. The *Nicomachean Ethics* compares knowing in moral matters to knowing in medicine and describes practical reasoning or phronesis as their characteristic virtue. In the process, practical reasoning is distinguished from wisdom and from scientific knowledge: inquiries into ethics and health, Aristotle writes, are particular, circumstantial, and therefore necessarily uncertain:

> The type of accounts we demand should reflect the subject matter, and questions about actions and expediency, like questions about health, have no fixed and invariable answers. And when our general account is so inexact, the account of particular cases is all the more inexact . . . and the agents themselves must consider in each case what the opportune action is.[4]

It is not that medicine and moral inquiry have no use for certainty or "fixed and invariable answers": nothing would make physicians or moral reasoners happier. But as objects of knowledge, health and morals differ from physical phenomena, about which certainty is available. For moral questions, as for questions about the care of patients, absolute or invariant answers are unobtainable. For this reason, scientific reasoning, or *episteme*, is inappropriate in fields like medicine, ethics, law, or meteorology, disciplines that are interpretive because they are radically uncertain. Episteme belongs, instead, to stable physical phenomena that can be known through necessary and invariant laws. Medicine and morals (like navigation, law, and meteorology) call for phronesis or practical reasoning, the ability to determine the best action to take in particular circumstances that cannot be distilled into universally applicable solutions. While scientific reasoning has precision and replicability as its goals, practical reasoning seeks the best answers possible under the circumstances. It enables the reasoner to distinguish, in a given situation, the better choice from the worse. The former is law-like and generalizable to every similar instance, while the latter is inescapably particular and interpretable, applicable to only a small set of more richly detailed circumstances.

Aristotle is not alone in describing a kind of thinking distinct from the rationality of science. Since the eighteenth century, the West has so privileged scientific reasoning that we in the twenty-first are still working free of the assumption that quantitative science is the only valid kind of knowing. Yet a number of thinkers have described another mode of knowing that in various ways resembles phronesis. William James described rationality as larger than scientific hypothesis and verification. "To say that all human thinking is essentially of two kinds—reasoning on the one hand, and narrative, descriptive, contemplative thinking on the other—is to say only what every reader's experience will corroborate," he wrote.[5] Hermeneutics, from Wilhelm Dilthey through Hans-Georg Gadamer, describes the interpretive circularity that characterizes the negotiation of a fit between general and particular. Not only has this view of knowing come to be recognized as the principal cognitive method in the qualitative social sciences and the humanities, but philosophers and sociologists of science have described its relevance to the physical sciences as well.[6] Pragmatism, too, from its originators, C. S. Peirce and William James, to Richard Rorty, has focused on what can practically be known rather than on attempting to locate the foundations of knowledge. A principle, John Dewey argued, is not an absolute truth but a hypothesis to be tested against the particularities of real-life circumstance.[7] About the failure to appreciate such nondeductive, practical reasoning, Hilary Putnam has observed: "The contemporary tendency to regard interpretation as something second class reflects . . . not a craving for objectivity but a craving for absolutes . . . and a tendency which is inseparable from that craving, the tendency to thinking that if the absolute is unobtainable, then 'anything goes.' " Against this bugbear of relativism he declares: "But enough is enough, enough isn't everything."[8]

In a number of social science fields, an appreciation of interpretive rationality has replaced earlier aspirations to become an exact science. Social and cultural anthropologists like Clifford Geertz and Stanley Tambiah borrowed the concept of interpretive rationality 30 years ago to move their discipline from its early scientism to an examination of its own methodology.[9] Similarly, historians abandoned mid-twentieth-century efforts to identify "laws" of history. Historiographers like Hayden White and Dominick La Capra have demonstrated instead the discipline's inescapably narrative construction of historical events and their significance.[10] The cognitive psychologist Jerome Bruner has given empirical teeth to these beliefs, arguing that the construction of narrative accounts is a fundamental way of thinking, even speculating that a desire to tell a story may underlie the acquisition of language in early childhood.[11] Nevertheless, in medicine—and often in the analytic philosophy that bioethics draws on—science continues to be the model for knowing. So pervasive is the misdescription of practical reason in Western culture that the philosopher Charles Taylor has argued that it warps contemporary attitudes toward rationality. If the "model of practical reasoning," he says, is "based on an illegitimate extrapolation from reasoning in natural science, little can meet its criteria and skepticism about reason itself is the consequence."[12]

Physicians use both the scientific or hypothetico-deductive and the practical or interpretive and narrative, but it is the latter that makes them clinicians. They rely, of course, on what biologists know and learn, for while medicine is not itself a science, it is undoubtedly a rational, science-using practice. Clinicians speak of their "knowledge base," but a better image comes from baseball. In medicine, scientific information acts as a kind of backstop for the physician's clinical reasoning. Ideas are pitched, and pathophysiology determines what remains in play. To be knowledgeable, a physician must keep up with the results of both scientific and clinical research and to add that information to the store of knowledge about the body, healthy and ill, through the study of human biology. More remains to be discovered in the biomedical sciences, and to some degree (more than with history, less than with chemistry) such knowledge is "fixed" and reliable.

Yet the very certainty that makes biology essential to medicine limits its usefulness in the care of patients. That use is never mere "application," and the relevance of any given scientific fact to a particular patient is always potentially uncertain.[13] Science generalizes and abstracts. Its rules have a timeless rigor, while patients, diseases, and therapeutic results are astonishingly, obstreperously variable. Even as clinical medicine aspires to the reliability of science, it must struggle to make sense of life's often unsorted particularities.

Scientific generalizations are useful for practical reasoning in medicine, but neither biological facts nor epidemiological probabilities go very far alone. In their approximate applicability, those general truths resemble legislative law or ethical principles. In the three professions that go back to the Middle Ages— law, moral theology, and medicine—generalizations require interpretation as they are put into action with particular people in varied, changing, or incompletely specified circumstances. These abstractions sometimes fit well, sometimes poorly, but never in detail. In fact, just to decide which general principle, law, or maxim is applicable to the present case, a reasoner must begin with a preliminary, provisional interpretation. The sound is a heart murmur or the bumps a rash. The situation is seen as one to which some generalization may apply. Is this patient's chest pain from heart or gut or chest muscles? Are these reddish bumps a contact rash or the beginning of measles? Deduction may decide the question—erythematous belly rashes in childhood are a sign of measles; this child has an erythematous belly rash and has not been immunized; therefore, this child almost certainly has measles. But the construction of the syllogism on which that deduction depends requires clinical judgment for both the recognition of the patient's symptoms or physical signs and the creation of the list of possibilities, the differential diagnosis. And that is a circular, narrative, interpretive undertaking.

Clinical Judgment as Narrative Rationality

Despite medicine's appeal to the canons of physical science as a model for its work, physicians do not reason as they imagine scientists do. Whether making a diagnosis, deciding on treatment, or working out the choices that have in the past 25 years come to be known as bioethics,[14] physicians when face to face with a patient do not proceed as they and their textbooks often describe it: top-down, deductively, "scientifically."[15] They use case-based reasoning instead.

Although the medical case is often regarded as a scientific report and even has been described as mere "patter," it is nevertheless a strongly conventional if minimalist narrative. Despite all the prohibitions against "anecdotal knowledge" in medicine, case narration is the principal means of thinking and remembering—of *knowing*—in medicine. The interpretive reasoning required to understand signs and symptoms and to reach a diagnosis is represented in all its situated and circumstantial uncertainty in narrative. This is not a quaint holdover from the pre-scientific past but rather the best means of representing the exercise of clinical judgment, medicine's phronesis. The practical reality of diagnosis and therapy—for chest pain, let's say—requires just such a flexible, situated, and reinterpretable means of representation. Physicians must know the facts of pathophysiology, the biological "laws," but they cannot start there. They start instead with the individual patient: the symptoms and signs and answers to questions that fill out the story of the illness presented to medical attention. The patient is a 43-year-old woman with radiating shoulder pain, chest discomfort, left arm weakness. Narrative accommodates far more variability than, say, the principles of human biology that describe the narrowing of coronary arteries. And it starts, where medicine must, with the odd details that sometimes go unrecognized as a heart attack. Narrative's sequential presentation unfolds the tactful, tactical deployment of knowledge and experience relevant to determining what is wrong with one particular patient and deciding what action to take on her behalf. Most important, case narrative supplies a workable medium for representing knowledge that is time- and context-dependent. Once the diagnosis is made, physicians may say, "Her story is consistent with a myocardial infarction."

Physicians share this narrative rationality with lawyers, moral reasoners, and detectives, all of whom must negotiate the fit between the organizing principles of their professional worldview and specific problematic situations. In each field, such a set of circumstances is called a "case." The rational procedure that determines what any particular given case is a case *of* is neither induction nor deduction but a third thing: the logic that the pragmatist C. S. Peirce described as "abduction" or "retroduction."[16] Reasoners start from a particular phenomenon and, using preliminary evidence, hypothesize its possible causes; those hypotheses are tested against details revealed by closer examination. This circular, interpretive procedure moves between generalities in the taxonomy of disease and particular signs and symptoms of the individual case until a workable conclusion is reached. Far from barring rules and generalities, narrative rationality—Peirce's "abduction"— puts them to interpretive work. Whether as history, a professional case, or the evening news, narrative provides a means by which the reasoner tests both intermediate moral formulations and ethical judgments (killing in self-defense, for example) and the general laws themselves ("Thou shalt not kill"), and it works out the implications in the concrete particulars of human lives.[17] So it is in medicine, where case narrative captures and represents clinical reasoning. Recorded in the chart and presented orally for teaching and review, the case is the template for a clinician's diagnostic thinking. It enables clinicians to consider the relevant abstractions—in this instance, the biological "plots" of disease mechanisms for possible diagnoses that can explain a 43-year-old woman's particular set of symptoms. Could a woman so young be having a heart attack? The received pathophysiological accounts of disease at once test clinical experience and are tested by it, both in the moment as the physician calls up analogous cases from a store of experience and later through the case presentations that make up the discourse of academic medicine. Cases are narratives created to organize, record, and think about practical experience.

Narrative, thus, is essential to thinking and knowing in clinical medicine. We take this rationality for granted, for we are narrative beings. Our lives are full of stories: we read and tell and listen to them; we watch them unfold in art, ritual, and social life; we perform them ourselves; they give form and meaning to our daily existence. We know ourselves as selves and as members and heirs of families, communities, and nations through the stories that exist about those collectivities and us. Recorded, recited, filmed, and whispered, narrative stores both memories of the past and visions of the future. Our lives are played out through and against them.

Narrative has been recognized, since at least Alasdair MacIntyre's *After Virtue*, as the individual's means of constructing and knowing the moral self.[18] But despite their particularity, narratives are not only individual. They are also communal, intersubjective, implicitly or overtly collaborative, and therefore conventional and audience-dependent. Even the most personal accounts—of courtship, for example, or chronic illness—take their shape from the body of tellable story forms, from plots and a shared sense of their importance and meaning.[19] They are a means of knowing others and of being known; they transmit knowledge in a community of practice and play a large part in creating and refining a moral or professional consensus. Whether narrative takes the form of fiction, history, life story, or gossip, culture and individual existence meet there.[20] Stories enable us to create and maintain our sense of self within our social and historical circumstances.

The function of narrative in clinical medicine is no different. There the construction and interpretation of stories—natural histories of disease, accounts of the patient's illness, clinical case narratives, diagnostic plots— enable physicians to make sense of circumstances and determine, even in situations of tragic choice, what, on the whole, is the best thing to do. Narrative, of course, is the antithesis of all that is believed to be scientific, and every physician knows it. As medical students, they learn to construct, record, and present cases—above all, to think with them—and at the same time they are taught a suspicion of anecdotal evidence, the singular occurrence that can skew perception. This only seems contradictory. Skepticism about narrative is an entirely justified, although sometimes myopically misunderstood, part of clinical rationality. Patrolling the borders of medical discourse, suspicion of the anecdote restrains medical narrative and blocks incursions of the irrelevant or the emotional. In the strictly conventional form of a medical case, narrative is still immersed in time, change, subjectivity, and contingency; the medical case both expresses and constrains these volatile qualities. They are the source of the value of the case—and its danger. Physicians must have a means of understanding and representing illness and disease that accommodates the knower's unabashedly situated subjectivity and the disease's entanglement with time. As the case orders events of the illness both chronologically and subjectively, it asserts or implies some causal relation among those events and imputes character and motive to the actors who are very nearly effaced.[21]

One of narrative's chief values for medicine lies exactly in the indeterminacy that makes it suspect. Even with the most linear, conventional, chronological plots—think of a recent explosive action film—the conclusion is never entirely predictable. As narrative depicts events embedded in the lives and concerns of its protagonists, circumstances unfold through time in all their contingency and complexity.[22] Endings may seem inevitable—but only after the fact. Whether a medical case, a person's life story, or a nation's political history, narrative explores the way cause and effect are entangled with the imponderables of human character and motivation, and with luck and happenstance.[23] Although the imponderable details may represent for the people involved what is most valued in a life or a history, those particularities are left behind as inessential whenever moral principles, clinical rules, or political generalizations are abstracted from events. Narrative, however, remains mired in the circumstances of human experience. From a scientific point of view, this is a weakness, but it is also narrative's practical strength. With the power implicit in designating particular details "facts" or occurrences "events," to say nothing of the persuasiveness of its use of rhetorical strategies in the representation of those facts and events, narrative constructs and interprets meaning. Whether as history or fiction or biography (an unstable amalgam of the first two) narrative captures experience and offers it vicariously to its readers and listeners, who not only learn from its explicit content but also absorb important lessons through the interpretive process of making sense of what they read or hear.[24]

In medicine, narrative is essential for the transfer of clinical knowledge and insight gained from practice. The clinical case history not only provides a means of working out and remembering what is best to do for a given patient but also captures experience and presents it to its audience. As a result, case narrative is the primary, vicarious means of shaping clinical judgment for new learners and experienced practitioners alike. Given the essentially moral character of clinical judgment—the intellectual virtue of determining what best to do for a sick patient—construction of the medical case is a specialized instance of narrative more generally: an essential means of moral knowing. As Stanley Hauerwas has described it, narrative represents events of moral importance as embedded in the lives and ongoing concerns of human beings; it is the means by which the meaning of deeds and lives is made known both to the actors themselves and to their community.[25] Diagnosis and treatment choice, thus, are not simply matters of logic or a patient preference exercised in the moment but a more contextual consideration intertwined with history, identity, culture, and the meaning of an individual's life. To make such a decision, practical reasoners draw upon information, experience, and desire and assess the present situation in their light.

In describing moral judgment, Aristotle held that experience was essential to phronesis, and therefore, he denied it to the young.[26] Internship and residency programs, from this point of view, are hothouses for the cultivation of

clinical judgment, and narrative is their essential medium. Not only is case
narrative the form taken by the physician's stock of clinical experience but
it also embodies the process of clinical reasoning that must become second
nature. This goes far to explain the suspicion with which individual assertions
of clinical judgment are regarded in the medical profession. Clinicians who
override the recommendations of residents with a declaration beginning "in
my clinical judgment" are almost always drawing on anecdotal experience
unmixed with published studies. Everyone knows that the single case is subjective, partial, likely to be skewed, and unrepresentative. It is even possibly
a singular irreplicable (although still never negligible) occurrence. Because
clinical education is organized to defeat such anecdotal bias, physicians learn
to scrutinize and excoriate the case narrative upon which they depend. Yet,
thanks to chance and to biological, clinical, and epidemiological research, the
borders of the narratable are always shifting. With the discovery of Legionnella, a new pneumonia could be discriminated; the standard account of the
presentation of heart disease has been refined to include the symptoms that
women experience. Medicine's clinical goal is to achieve skeletal diagnostic
plots and boring treatment protocols—which feel quite scientific—for every
disease and for the choice and conduct of their treatment. Yet case narrative
has not disappeared from medicine or medical education, nor is it likely
to. Outliers exist, and in clinical practice they are inescapably important. A
middle-class 30-year-old woman presents with all the symptoms of scurvy,
and a history of bulimia is discovered; a 20-year-old's iron deficiency anemia
turns out to be caused by celiac sprue. In every case, even those that are well
settled and blessedly ordinary, the patient first must be diagnosed, and this
will always be the interpretive task for a well-informed, skilled observer.

The narrative character of clinical knowledge owes its tenacity in an era
of scientific medicine to the profession's duty to make sense of the signs and
symptoms of illness in every particular patient. With a grasp of human biology,
clinical epidemiology, and medical decision-making, a physician is, above
all, as Stephen Toulmin has pointed out, the person who takes the patient's
history—and, he might have added, transforms it into a medical case.[27] At
its richest and most skilled, this act of narrative perception and construction
requires the capacity to understand the patient and recast his or her story
of illness into a medical narrative that can be matched with the diagnostic
taxonomy and lead to appropriate treatment. Case narrative draws on several
clinical abilities: the elicitation of useful information from the patient, the
performance of a good physical examination, a focused and parsimonious
use of tests, the prescription of efficacious therapy with minimal harm to
the patient, and attention to the psychological, moral, and social problems

that may arise in connection with the illness and its treatment. The clinical judgment these tasks require is not science or scientific reasoning but practical, interpretive reasoning, the exercise of phronesis.

An Education for Clinical Judgment

The education meant to cultivate phronesis or clinical judgment in future physicians replicates medicine's complex negotiation between biological science and particular experience with patients. The first two years of medical school, years of intensive study of human biology, are merely preliminary. The third and fourth years are spent, first, observing the clinical use of scientific information in the diagnosis and treatment of the seriously ill and, then, gradually, under guidance, assuming some of the responsibilities of patient care. Third-year students have the unstated task of working out how science fits with clinical phenomena and how it is used in practical reasoning. As they recast the biology they have spent years learning into clinically relevant cases, they move toward the acquisition of clinical judgment. It is a confusing time, and clinical teachers are regularly heard complaining that, while their apprentices may be the cream of the educational crop, they don't seem to know very much at all. Yet, as students participate in the care of patients and construct the cases that are part of that care, they learn very quickly. They spend their days in the hospital interpreting not from science to disease or from clinical generalizations to the patient's symptoms but the other (and at first confusing) way around: from symptoms to diagnosis and then, if necessary, to the science.

The principal tool in this process, both for students learning clinical reasoning and for the experts teaching them, is the case. It organizes clinical observation and investigation and models the analogical process by which clinical reasoners reach a recognizable diagnosis.[28] Students learn classic descriptions of diseases, their standard presentations or "disease pictures," and then go on to gather cases that illustrate variations in presenting symptoms, timing and course of illness, therapeutic response, and outcome. In the process, "disease pictures" become a sequence of stills, then take on the flow of a film—ready for editing (to continue the metaphor), with alternate scenes and optional endings. The basic plot, however, is clear, and medicine's work is to intervene to shorten it and, if possible, give it a happy ending.

Students write up cases in patients' charts (hence third-year "clerkships"), present them orally to instructors, and soon adopt them as their mental template for inquiry and recollection. As they gather details, students begin to make medical sense of patients' signs and symptoms and to construct, record, and report their case histories. In this, they resemble naturalists rather than laboratory scientists. Starting as nearly as possible from the beginning with each patient, they observe—experience—the evidence firsthand and put it together with only conditional certainty. They construct professionally acceptable narrative accounts of what they observe and learn which normal findings to include and which to exclude in order to buttress their reasoning. They take time to invoke biological science for explanation only when the clinical details do not fit a well-known pattern or when they have a teacher who demands it. By means of this clinical method, they begin to acquire the rudiments of clinical judgment, and in the process they learn to be skeptical of every sort of information, a skepticism that is integral to medicine's practical rationality.

Two years of such experience with individual patients and constant review by more experienced practitioners produce graduates who are well versed in the observation and formulation of cases. As residents, depending on the specialty they choose, they will spend three to five more years accumulating experience in this interpretive activity, gradually assuming responsibility for the diagnosis and treatment of patients. Each new physician acquires and sorts the taxonomy of medical case knowledge by observing clinical phenomena and their alteration over time. Chief among their discoveries is the lesson that, although much in diagnosis and treatment is replicable and therefore predictable, much is not. Diagnosis requires a retrospective reconstruction of events; every treatment is to some degree experimental. Even the most reliable patient with clear-cut symptoms is a potentially uncertain field of knowledge. Physicians understand this and rely on their store of knowledge and experience and on the rational method inherent in the construction of the case. They are not scientists or artists but practical reasoners, exercising clinical judgment as they see patients and work out what ought to be done for each one them.

Clinical education is thus finely calibrated to instill and reward the development of clinical judgment in the face of uncertainty.[29] Although it bears little resemblance to the cool and objective, positivist ideal of physical science that it takes as it model, this practical rationality, the physician's exercise of clinical judgment, is likely to be taken as evidence for medicine's status as a science. As students improve their construction and presentation of clinical cases, they absorb the lesson that they are expected to be meticulous and thorough. "Science" is the goad that urges them on to perfection, and the skepticism they absorb confirms them in this stance. But there is no need for physicians to borrow these qualities from science. Thoroughness and skepticism are also the property of thinkers as diverse as historians and literary critics. They are virtues that also belong to the profession of medicine.

Meanwhile, the goal of medical education is clinical judgment: the interpretive tact or educated common sense that sometimes rises to intuitive insight, even genius, when exercised by a master clinician in the diagnosis and treatment of a person who is ill.[30] Neither science nor art, it is an intellectual capacity carefully cultivated through the rigors of a long apprenticeship spent dealing with radical uncertainty. It is clinical judgment. Such ability in clinical knowing is held to be the crowning quality of the expert clinician—and, as often as not, by the very same physicians who claim that medicine is itself a science. Neither book-learning nor simple experience, clinical judgment is the *je ne sais quoi* of medical practice. Physician-educators disagree about how to teach it; they even debate whether it might not be innate and unteachable. Still, during the long clinical apprenticeship designed to inculcate it, individual professors feel perfectly able to say which of the young physicians in their charge possess it and to what degree. Residents are likely to resent it as a power play—"in my clinical judgment"—used by elders who do not have recently published clinical studies or the strategies of evidence-based medicine at their fingertips. But in the absence of certain knowledge about the individual case, the goal of their professional education remains the development of good clinical judgment. It is this that will enable them to do their best for particular patients one by one.

PART II

Clinical Judgment and the Idea of Cause

CHAPTER FOUR

⌒

"What Brings You Here Today?": The Idea of Cause in Medical Practice

> Sergeant Lewis: "They don't make any sense."
> Morse: "Things never do until you find out."
>
> —COLIN DEXTER

MY DAUGHTER'S ILLNESS sent me on a quest to understand the idea of cause. To know the cause of disease is to have control. Medicine is driven by it, and patients and their families are part of that drive. And yet, as I discovered, the idea of cause in medical practice bears as odd a relation to science as clinical medicine itself. The physician's investigation of cause, even as it seems to confirm clinical medicine's status as a science, undercuts that claim at every turn.

The idea of cause fits right into the misdescription of medicine because it is central to the profession's conventional, positivist ideal of science. Yet in the physician's office or the emergency room, cause is the object of a retrospective, narrative investigation that more nearly resembles investigation in history or economics than experiments in microbiology or chemistry. The face-to-face encounter with a patient gives what the physician knows about biological cause a practical, taken-for-granted, confirmatory role. What science has yet to discover seldom comes to mind—and then only in truly puzzling cases. Physicians instead are in pursuit of a diagnosis, the cause of the patient's illness, and this causal pursuit is framed as science rather than as simply a rational inquiry. Yet a look at the clinical uses of cause reveals some of the important ways clinical medicine differs from a Newtonian science and highlights instead medicine's practical rationality, the clinical judgment essential to the work of diagnosis and treatment. At the same time, the importance of clinical cause suggests why physicians might claim the label "science" for their work and why that label goes unquestioned both in medicine and out.

Clinical Cause

Physicians are concerned with clinical cause, and since questions of cause are essential to the sciences, that concern is assumed to guarantee medicine's status as science.[1] Explanation is what science is all about. What is the structure of the universe, the means by which it works? Or the body, its organs, its DNA? Hypotheses are generated, variables controlled, experiments conducted, results analyzed; knowledge is elaborated, revised, advanced. This powerful method characterizes much of biomedical research and is readily understood as the investigation of cause. What causes cancer? Or AIDS? Or tuberculosis? These are scientific questions about the chain of events leading to an unexpected lump or night sweats or a cough that physicians recognize as disease. Biomedical scientists work to understand some part of these causal chains well enough to suggest how they might be interrupted or altered. Their goal is to change the outcome so the disease can be cured or, better yet, prevented.

When we are ill, we go to a doctor to find out why. We want to know the cause and expect that science will supply the answer. What could be more scientific? Yet, while biology plays an essential role in clinical medicine, the idea of cause in medical practice is a far simpler, narrower concern. In clinical medicine, especially academic medicine, cause is that without which a subsequent effect would not occur: Aristotle's efficient cause.[2] The idea can encompass a long chain of circumstance: someone sneezes, covers her face, and not long afterward shakes hands with a friend, who turns to pick up a sandwich; the virus binds to the friend's respiratory epithelium; cells receive the signal to replicate and thrive in adjacent cells, provoking an inflammatory response: mucus membranes swell, body temperature rises; the friend has chills, muscle aches: he is sick and cancels his plans for tomorrow. This is complicated in its detail, but it is nevertheless simple and strongly linear. First one thing happens, then as its consequence another. Physicians know a multitude of these causal sequences. They make up the clinical plots of hundreds of maladies and their variants. Well established in pathophysiology, these sequences are sorted into the taxonomy of disease that physicians rely on when they set out to make sense of a patient's symptoms. Biomedical science supplies the information that shapes these accounts of disease, and the knowledge of that science grounds the diagnostic expertise that prompts people who are sick to seek medical attention. Yet the addition of science to medicine little more than a century ago, while it enormously expanded information, did not much alter the procedures of clinical thinking. The way physicians reasoned before the scientific era is, in its broad outlines, the way they reason today.[3]

The clinical encounter focuses on a pressing, practical question: What is causing this particular patient to feel ill? This is the question of clinical cause, a more specific and targeted causal question than either the biological problem of disease etiology or the more contingent, multiplicative question of how one particular person fell ill. Both biological cause and the puzzle of individual etiology have a role to play in medical practice. But this more limited, everyday idea—half of "cause and effect"—is the concept of cause used by physicians in the care of patients and assumed throughout medical education. Its primacy is unquestioned by physicians even as they describe their work as science. Arising later in the causal trajectory, it concerns the identity of the malady rather than its scientific explanation or the history of its particular development in a single patient. Those other causal concepts are subordinated to the goal that is the sine qua non of patient care: the reliable determination of a diagnosis.[4]

This down-home, practical idea of cause seems to support the belief that medicine is a science. Simple and linear, clinical cause fits the conventional physics-based vision of science that physicians invoke as their professional ideal. And for physicians, medical practice may actually feel like science. As they work toward solving the problem of clinical cause, they hope to reduce it to a taken-for-granted invisibility. Because clinicians are immersed in unpredictable circumstances, they often must respond experimentally, using their best guesses and watching for confirmation or failure. They use the scientific strategy of isolating or focusing on the minimal unit—the lungs or the pulmonary function tests—in a way that now seems obviously scientific. It produces good results, and when things go well, their exercise of clinical judgment is satisfyingly linear. Diagnostic hypotheses are ventured, focused and refined, then confirmed. Practical reasoning proceeds normally, habitually, and as if automatically for the well-informed physician. If the patient's condition is recognizable, the question of cause all but disappears. It shrinks to something like a professional reflex or tacit knowledge, as decisions are made and action taken in accord with well-established practice.[5]

At times, however, when the diagnosis is uncertain or therapy lacks a clear indication, clinical reasoning becomes patent. Then it is visibly multiplicative and nonlinear, and its procedures themselves become the object of clinical scrutiny. Clinical skepticism calls into question the routine grasp of biological laws and evokes a more speculative and potentially complex causality. Although clinical method remains the same, it widens to become more obviously contextual, as remotely plausible hypotheses are generated and engaged. Then, at moments when medicine is most uncertain, physicians are most nearly like the scientists they idealize. Then they "think outside the box": they question received knowledge, open themselves to new possibilities, propose experiments. At such times, belief in the reliability of clinical knowledge is provisionally suspended, and medicine spreads its narrative net to catch the unexpected contributory factor or an odd correlate, the telling detail, a predisposition or risk factor. This means that, while physicians may profess a simple, linear idea of cause and effect, they frequently work as if cause were complex and multifaceted.

The idea of cause in clinical medicine is thus both taken-for-grantedly simple and ambiguously multiplicative—and each by turns as the situation requires. These two concepts are not at all alike. One is the linear idea of ordered, necessary, and sufficient biological causality, the concept physicians always hope to rely upon. The other is a more complex, multilevel speculative and narrative assumption that comes to the fore at need. The two concepts of cause exist side by side in medical practice. The linear "mechanisms of disease" and the richer, more circumstantial and contingent idea of cause do not harmonize or reconcile, but neither are they doomed to conflict. When cause can be simplified, it is taken for granted: clinical practice is understood to be science, and cause tends to disappear from the experienced reasoner's consciousness. When cause cannot be simplified, the problem is represented and examined as a hypothetical narrative of an unsolved case. This difference between medicine's simple causal norm and its frequently more complex reality is ignored. Obscured by the visual field defect in the profession's understanding of its knowledge, the oddity does not even come to consciousness as justification when—as I will show in later chapters—physicians regularly, usefully, and on principle ignore the implications of the science claim.

Meanwhile, in the examination room, physicians address the question of cause in a distinctive way. Linear causation, while it satisfies medicine's positivist ideal, is not quite the pillar of clinical method it might seem. This is because the patient poses the problem of cause in reverse: not as cause-and-effect but the other way around. Effects are manifest in the patient's body; what has caused them? Diagnosis requires a retrospective understanding of the events of illness. What has gone wrong in this patient's body? What has occasioned the signs and symptoms of illness in this particular person? Where in the chain of causation will it be possible to intervene so as to alter the ill effects and cure or ameliorate the malady? These clinical questions are posed backward, from effect to cause, and the data required to answer them come initially from the patient's account of illness. It is not that the physician's questions are unscientific but that, in answering them, biology and epidemiology are the factual givens rather than the objects of diagnostic investigation. The clinical inquiry is an interpretive quest that circles between biology and epidemiology on the one hand and the circumstantial details of the patient's presentation of the symptoms and clinical signs of illness on the other. Biology and epidemiology are matters of secondary, instrumental interest. They will be important, one mapped upon the other, in determining what is the matter with the patient, but they are not themselves in question. In taking care of patients, the important causal question for physicians is the clinical one they are called upon to answer dozens of times a day: What is causing this patient's symptoms?

This is a narrower, interpretive question, and to answer it, physicians use both scientific knowledge and information about individual cause supplied by epidemiology and clinical research as tools in the retrospective narrative reconstruction of events. The tools are not themselves investigated. Thus, clinical cause is best understood as a narrative hypothesis rather than a scientific one, and narratively and historically is exactly how, as a practical matter, physicians explore the causal question that most concerns them. After taking the patient's history, they ask about symptoms and then examine the patient for signs in order to construct a recognizable clinical account of the patient's illness. Biology and what is known of the etiology of disease enable them to transform details of the patient's illness narrative into clues that will match one disease plot better than others and clinch the diagnosis. But this inquiry has nothing to do with an interest in scientific cause or the description of the causal chain in this particular case. If physicians are able now and then to add to the stock of biological knowledge or to the clinical understanding of disease etiology, so much the better. But their primary task, their professional duty, lies elsewhere. The cause of the patient's symptoms is the cause that the medical profession exists to identify and treat. Once that cause is determined, the malady will look as simple and straightforward as a textbook account. In retrospect, illness events will fall predictably into line. But precisely because clinical inquiry proceeds backward in relative ignorance into the life experience of the patient, discovery of the cause of a patient's illness is not a simple or a linear task.

Opening Questions

"What brings you here today?"

The clinical encounter of patient and physician begins with a question about cause: the motive for the patient's being there, some reason for interrupting an everyday routine, or the impetus that has propelled this person into the bright light of medical scrutiny. But here, as elsewhere in clinical practice (and unlike its simple, positivist ideal), cause is complicated and not reliably linear. Physicians are well aware that illness is neither a necessary nor a sufficient condition for making a doctor's appointment. Some diseases lack symptoms; other maladies impair so slowly that the loss of function, especially past middle age, seems normal. At every age, the "worried well" present themselves for reassurance, while other people in serious pain delay seeing a doctor. And almost every physician can tell a story of a patient who has glared back suspiciously and said: "That's what I'm here for you to find out," or has answered—right out of vaudeville but truthfully enough—"My wife."

Still, the physician's opening question is a useful one. Patients are likely to answer with the symptom that most troubles them. In the language of medicine this is the "chief complaint": "I'm having terrible headaches" or "There's a lump here in my neck I need you to look at." Although they know that medicine aims to intervene in a chain of cause and effect so as to alter outcome, and they go to the doctor to reap the benefits of science and medical technology, sometimes with quite specific tests or therapies in mind, patients nevertheless are unlikely to answer "science."

For science is only a part of what patients expect. They come to the doctor, above all, just as the expression has it, seeking medical attention. If it's not a routine checkup, and sometimes when it is, the answer to the opening question is a symptom or a worry.[6] In the questions that follow, the physician will elicit further details that can explain the symptoms by locating them in the clinical taxonomy of disease. This explanation is what patients come for: not pathophysiological information but an interpretation of their malaise, the physician's judgment based on cumulative experience of this particular concatenation of biological events. Patients look for understanding in its several senses, for reassurance, and, often, for a prescription. They want to know what is going on with them and what to do about it. They want the physician to grasp how they are affected and to make sense of their illness in a way that in turn will make sense to them. Even a broken arm, that exemplum of a malady without much illness, needs this sort of attention. If it's summer and the young patient is in the midst of swimming lessons, she needs not only to have the bone set but also to be given a cast that is submersible. And if the malady is serious or requires life-altering treatment, patients want the physician to acknowledge the predicament they are in and to offer help and reassurance that the prescribed therapy is the best course to take. To paraphrase the old saying, patients hope for cure if possible, relief of suffering in any case, but comfort above all.

Medical attention is more than science, and certainly it differs from science as medicine customarily portrays it. Biological cause plays a strong part in medical care but an odd one: supremely useful, but taken for granted; complex and multiplicative, but regarded as if it were a row of dominoes. For the clinician, the original or formal scientific cause is not immediately pressing; it is not even at that moment very interesting. As fascinating as the question of scientific cause may be in and of itself, especially for a new disease or an old one newly explained, in the normal discourse of clinical medicine, etiology is important chiefly as a part of the method for determining what is wrong with the patient.[7] Because etiology traces the necessary, if perhaps not sufficient, cause of symptoms that are the primary concern in a clinical encounter, knowledge of that etiology functions diagnostically as a given. The more immediate problem posed by the patient's symptoms is the limited causal question of diagnosis. As a result, because a good diagnosis is central to good medical care, scientific causality is flattened, and the clinical reasoner, if asked, is likely to report that really there isn't any science involved. It's only a matter of understanding what is going on, she may say; just common sense.[8] The question of cause has disappeared into its givenness for this knower in this particular case.

"Any foreign travel?" To make the diagnosis, physicians elicit clues by asking questions that are understood to be implicitly causal: "What did he have to eat?" "What sort of work do you do?" These are questions about individual cause as it maps onto known etiologies. They attempt to establish quasi-causal details, necessary if not sufficient,[9] that can explain the illness the patient is presenting for diagnosis. Every disease has a "natural history," and physicians during their clinical training absorb as many of them as memory can possibly hold. Often described as the recognition of "disease pictures," diagnosis is more like recognizing a movie from a photographic "still" or a song from its opening notes. Diseases are narratives with recognizable variations unfolding over time. Like other narratives, they are typed and categorized until familiarity reduces them to a representative scene. Infectious, autoimmune, metabolic, vascular, neoplastic, genetic: the list is just a first cut at diagnostic typology, and each genre has subspecies characterized by variations in plot. In addition to the discriminative details of the patient's symptoms—a slow rather than a sudden onset, for example, or pain that is dull rather than stabbing—the events of the patient's life may suggest a likely diagnosis: the illness of family members, intravenous drug use, 20 years' work in a chemical plant, a visit to a region known for cholera, a recent vacation that ended with a celebrative dinner of barracuda steak. Given a well-established element in the natural history of a disease, its traces in the patient's narrative of illness serve as classificatory signs. Even if the diagnosis is not definite, its genre may be recognizable. Like Victorian turrets beneath a cloud-draped moon, the details of illness, its signs and symptoms, reveal to a clinical audience the kind of situation it is and what is likely to happen next. "Anyone in the family ill?" "Was he wearing a seat belt?" "When did the fever start?"

Narrative accounts of disease mechanisms or pathophysiological processes are the principal means of organizing symptomatic clues and their interpretive syndromes. Established by biological and epidemiological research, these causal narratives are memorized in medical school and are readily available in medical textbooks. Physicians reason abductively, backward from signs and symptomatic effects to the diseases that may be their cause. Those etiologic plots—sudden onset of pain, say, followed by nausea with fever and chills— supply patterns of timing and detail that function as narrative criteria that, if the diagnosis is correct, the patient's malady can be expected to fulfill. Unlike laboratory science, which is free to use the building blocks of others' investigation, this clinical retrospection calls for the physician's firsthand knowledge of the patient's illness—not simply as a moral obligation but as an essential part of clinical reasoning.[10] Jerome Groopman describes it this way:

> In having him repeat his medical history and physical examination now for the fourth time, I wasn't merely performing a perfunctory ritual. . . . If I were to care for him properly, first I had to confirm the accuracy of the information abstracted in his records. And even if I discovered no new fact or physical finding, there was a journey taken when I listened to a patient recount his story and I palpated his body. It was a journey of the senses—hearing, touching, seeing—that carried me to the extra-sensory dimension of intuition.[11]

Physicians ask about the onset of the present illness and the duration and intensity of its symptoms; they examine the patient's body for signs of disease and, if needed, order tests. They match the details of this particular illness against more general patterns ranged in the taxonomy of disease as they circle from particular detail to general description and back again, gathering additional data with more precisely focused questions and tests. Focus comes with experience, but even in young physicians it can be honed and made more explicit with the knowledge of clinical epidemiology and the strategies of medical decision-making.[12] Thus the pathophysiologic details of scientific etiology and the Bayesian inferences about the probability of disease in patients of particular descriptions take their place as givens by which an illness is understood.[13] The result is a list of diagnostic possibilities, the differential diagnosis. The next clinical task is the only clear occasion for deduction in clinical medicine: ruling in or ruling out the diagnostic possibilities, often with tests, until a match is found.

Diagnostic interpretation is the central act of clinical knowing. The physician's task is to decide in medical terms what has brought the patient here today. The pathophysiological mechanisms of disease are not the object of investigation in the clinical encounter, nor, beyond the diagnostic clues in the patient's history, is individual etiology a concern. It's not that biological cause and individual etiology are not important. That's clearly not the case. But they are not in question. At this moment, they are the givens, the facts, whose value for the clinician lies primarily in the clues they provide for diagnosis and occasionally in the possibilities they suggest for future prevention. If the patient is likely to get sick again (as with a diabetic in insulin crisis) pathophysiological causation may be discussed. An explanation of the way the pancreas malfunctions may persuade the patient to adhere to dietary restrictions or, farther along the causal chain, to follow a glucose-testing regimen more carefully.

The physician's narrow causal focus fits with the patient's concerns. For people who are ill, the pathophysiological cause of the malady takes a back seat to the clinical cause. People go to the doctor to learn what their symptoms mean and what should be done about them. The pathophysiological details are, for the moment and ultimately, irrelevant. Patients want to know what is wrong, if it's serious, how long it will last, whether it will alter their life plans. These questions have brought them to the doctor on this particular day. The symptoms may have persisted for weeks, but now, today, the patient wants a physician's interpretation of them. Some patients do want to understand the etiology of their disease: the slow accumulation of plaque that has narrowed and closed the artery, the mutation of the influenza virus that enables it to elude earlier immunities, or the body's failure to suppress a cell gone wild. When Michael Bérubé reports seeing a nurse's note in his son's chart, "Parents are intellectualizing," his wife responds, "That seems about right."[14] Others want only to know that their condition is recognizable to the physician. Almost without exception, however, all patients need a name for what ails them—the clinical cause—even if it turns out to be dire. To learn that they have a recognizable disease, even a life-defining one, is less upsetting for many people than to suspect it. "Just having a diagnosis," one patient said, "means the rest of your life can start." To the degree that a treatment is well established and efficacious, the mere act of naming a disorder can be comforting. For the physician not to identify the malady—even when the physical suffering is relieved or cured—is somehow disquieting, a source of unease in itself. Worst of all is to be told without explanation that "it's nothing; it's all in your head."

Diagnosis not only names the malady but also implies that it has a recognizable and therefore respectable cause. This is a principal reason people
with fibromyalgia or chronic fatigue syndrome struggle to have their maladies
named. A diagnostic label designates what is normal in the realm of the illness,
entails the treatment a patient can expect to be offered, and suggests the likely
outcome. Since many diagnostic labels have well-established social meanings,
some of this information is already in the patient's possession. Such meanings
are stored and transmitted in patients' stories of symptoms and therapy, danger
and recovery, disability or death. These social accounts of treated disease relate
what particular people have experienced and suggest that such experience is
common—or if not, then probable or within the realm of possibility. Everyone knows the diabetes story, the splotch-that-turned-out-to-be-melanoma
story, the walking-pneumonia story. Can this illness be subsumed under such
a heading? Will *this* case turn out to be like that? Physicians rely on these
common accounts (and sometimes must work to correct them) when they
diagnose and prescribe and prognosticate. Here scientific cause can be immediately useful in patient care. Although a pathophysiological disquisition—
especially one untranslated from medical texts or recent studies—is not the
explanation the patient needs, a good description of the way the relevant body
parts have been (or will be) affected can play a valuable part of making room
in the patient's world for the diagnosis that means an altered life course. For
patients as well as physicians, knowledge of scientific cause is a good substitute
for control.

The knowledge of scientific cause also allows the physician to display a
trustworthy expertise and to reinforce the necessity of following treatment
recommendations. This is especially important if the malady is new or strange.
When an upper respiratory infection is probably mycoplasma pneumonia,
caused by a life-form that is neither a bacterium nor a virus, the treatment
commonly prescribed can safely be stopped if it upsets the patient's stomach.
Accustomed to taking all of a prescribed antibiotic, the patient may need at
least a brief microbiological explanation in order to believe that in this instance
it is safe to discontinue the medicine. Causal explanation is also needed when
the etiologic story long associated with a set of symptoms has been proven
wrong. Someone with peptic ulcer disease these days may need to know its
scientific cause to be persuaded that this is not her father's peptic ulcer, a
condition that was attributed entirely to stress. The surprising discovery of
bacteria in what was once believed to be the sterile, acid-scoured stomach
means the patient will escape those bland white meals of milk and potatoes
that previous generations endured. There will be no surgery and no advice (or
in the United States maybe just a little) about stress management. Antibiotics

offer a cure, and it matters a lot—scientifically—that all the medicine is taken. Understanding the newly established etiology will help the patient trust the treatment and stick to it.

For most office visits, however, both scientific and individual cause are marginalized. They are fixed and unexplored as givens. This does not undermine the physician's opening question. What brings the patient to the doctor today is never understood to be a matter of disease etiology or part of an investigation of disease causality. Despite its ring of scientific investigation, the opening question is just what most patients take it to be: an inquiry meant to locate this visit first in a larger field of personal history and then in one of the pigeonholes of disease taxonomy. Its focused request for information is the starting point of a rational, retrospective, medical inquiry rather than a biological one.

For if medicine is not a science, it nevertheless is rigorously rational. The question that opens the patient-physician encounter begins a narrative, interpretive investigation as logical as any laboratory experiment. The difference is that physicians of necessity are retrospective practical reasoners who must test their hypotheses with the very data out of which they are formed.[15] No wonder they want firsthand knowledge! As medical informatics confirms, they cannot diagnose reliably from a secondhand report or even from a patient's test results.[16] More than cost prevents patients from being run through a body scanner upon entering a doctor's office. Pure induction, even the induction of the routine "complete physical," is almost always a waste of time. As Marsden Scott Blois argued in his early book on medical informatics, the patient's presenting complaint is essential to clinical reasoning because it constitutes an initial narrowing of the world of possibility, a focus that no computerized diagnostic program could operate without or (more important) generate on its own.[17] Physicians need a clue to begin a line of inquiry, and the symptom or concern that answers their opening question provides it: chest pain or a lump or insomnia. Recorded in the chart as the patient's chief complaint, this problem sets the agenda; the clinician's assumption is that it will point backward in time toward its cause, the diagnosis in question.

Often the cause will turn out to be interestingly different from that suggested by the symptom presented as the entrance ticket. Chest pain will turn out to be grief for a friend's death; sleeplessness will prompt a discussion of depression and perhaps some advice about alcohol consumption. The answer to the physician's opening question, nevertheless, is important. Even if the patient's presenting symptom is a red herring or the most minor detail of a complicated condition, but especially if it turns out to be unsupported by the test results, it needs to be addressed before the visit is over. The patient's answer to the opening question will not only go a long way toward shaping the physician's inquiry but also, to varying degrees, will guide the treatment. Beyond supplying pathophysiological clues, what brings the patient here to-day suggests something of the patient's character and circumstances and what will be needed for a successful use of biology, pharmacology, and clinical persuasion in this case.

Taken together, the questions and answers that open the clinical encounter declare a willingness on both sides to undertake the process of investigation, clinical interpretation, and amelioration. Knowledge that, for example, my-coplasma is caused by a prion, an intermediate form of biological life, or that peptic ulcers are the result of *helicobacter pylori* that can thrive in the otherwise sterile stomach we owe to scientific research.[18] But what goes on between doctors and patients with mycoplasma pneumonia or peptic ulcer disease is not science, not biology, but medicine. The opening question—"What brings you here today?" or the consultants' variant "What seems to be the trouble?" and the more recent faintly mercantile "What can I do for you?"—are not only the first lines of an interpretive investigation but also what may be the beginning of a new chapter in the patient's life. Question and reply constitute a human exchange that recognizes the patient's need and offers help. The interaction is undergirded by a moral commitment so strong that where it is limited or does not operate—as with physical examinations for employment or insurance, military or professional sports-team physicians, and now in some health maintenance organizations—the physician has a duty to be sure those patients know its limits. The patient-physician relationship is central to the professional privilege that medicine shares with law and the clergy, and its opening exchange is the starting point for the physician's retrospective narra-tive reconstruction of what is going on—individually, scientifically, but most of all clinically—in this particular case.

As the guarantor of disease etiology, then, scientific cause has an odd place in clinical medicine, at once powerfully useful and all but ignored. Important rhetorically with patients and a mark of the scientific (and thus the authoritative), the physician's knowledge of disease causality is central to everyday clinical practice. But this is for medical rather than for scientific reasons. While not the object of inquiry itself, such knowledge shapes the inaugural exchange between patient and physician, an encounter in which the question of cause is necessarily broader than the pathophysiological question of disease etiology. The physician's knowledge of scientific mechanisms and clinical etiology guides diagnostic interpretation, influences treatment, and provides reassurance to the patient. But throughout the patient-physician encounter, scientific questions are decentered and deferred. They merge with wider, more circumstantial considerations of illness in the individual. Once it is diagnosed and an appropriate treatment identified, the malady will seem very like the linear, cause-to-effect description found in textbooks, and its occurrence in this particular patient will (probably) fit what is known about it statistically. Until then, however, the patient's answer to the opening question—what brings her here today—and the medical interpretation the physician will begin to construct from the answer will be a contingent, multivariant narrative.

CHAPTER FIVE

⌐⌐

The Simplification of Clinical Cause

Compared with this world of living individualized feeling,
the world of generalized objects which the intellect
contemplates is without solidity or life.

—WILLIAM JAMES

MEDICINE STRIVES FOR causal simplicity. Its identification with the old-fashioned idea of science owes its strength to the straightforward cause-and-effect simplicity that physicians find there. They admire that simplicity and, although their practice—for good reason—often belies it, they have adopted it as a goal. And no wonder: the promise of ready diagnoses with safe and efficacious treatment draws young people to medical careers—to say nothing of bringing patients to physicians. Anomalies are intellectually interesting; their discovery may be the highlight of a good clinician's day—or career. But the goal of both clinical medicine and laboratory research is to understand and resolve them; discovery is important only as a first step toward their eventual renormalizing explanation. They are "resorbed," as clinicians say, back into the unremarkably ordinary. Thus, linear causality comes to stand for the clinical competence, the automaticity of thought, and the ready solutions to difficult problems that physicians work toward. When life or health is at risk, who does not want a what-you-see-is-what-you-get account of reality, a representation of things as they truly are, without distortion or bias?

The Simplification of Complexity

The simple, linear causality associated with the conventional idea of science seems to be just what it takes to diagnose and treat patients successfully. Not only does medicine's commitment to identifying and treating the patient's illness confirm the profession's self-conception as a science, but so compelling is the goal of acting on the patient's behalf that it flattens and simplifies everything in its way. What physicians know about complex cause in biology and the contingent status of knowledge in physics, their accumulated insights into the human condition, individual psychology, and social complexity—let alone any shred of contemporary philosophy of science—are all submerged. In their place, physicians develop a clinical skepticism and, its corollary, the obligation to know firsthand the imprecise evidence they must work with: the history of the patient's illness, the clinical symptoms and signs, the test results. Despite the welter of detail and the occurrence of anomalies and outliers so frequent as to threaten a sense of a stable diagnostic taxonomy, the clinical ideal remains simplicity, a straight line from cause to effect. The goal is the identification of the patient's malady: a convincing diagnosis and a clear choice of treatment.

This ideal is regularly challenged in everyday clinical medicine. Causal simplicity is never easy for medicine to achieve because the information it needs is social and circumstantial as well as scientific. Not only does the knowledge drawn from the minutely detailed, complex subdisciplines of biology come in overwhelming amounts, but the objects of biological investigation, unlike those of physics and chemistry, are (or once were) living beings. As a consequence, biology is multileveled and more contingent than the physical sciences.[1] Its imprecision is far greater than the indeterminacy of physics, where (as every premed student learns) observation becomes more limited in scope as it increases in precision and the observer unavoidably disturbs the observational field. Biological imprecision is even more thoroughgoing. Because living beings are harder to pin down than nonliving matter, variables are far less easily identified and controlled. And human biology is still more complicated because its objects have reasons as well as causes for their behavior. As a consequence, medicine must take account of cultural, social, familial, psychological details. Little wonder that David Morris has called illness biocultural.[2]

Seen in a systems-theory progression from microbe to cultural context, biomedical science is even more complex than the rest of biology, even less capable of certainty, because illness exists on so many levels.[3] Medical events and conditions can be described as cellular, organic, organismic, personal, familial, and cultural, and their causes can be too. What's more, cause runs both ways on the scale from cell to society since illness behavior is also social behavior, and microbial activity often depends upon it. Think of the spread of HIV or the annual subspeciation of influenza or *Legionnella* pneumonia. These patterns are objects of research, of course, but the investigation is dependent on such ill-controlled variables as sexual practices, international travel, and rooftop air-conditioning towers. These diachronic, multilevel aspects of illness render the question of cause in human illness more complex and contingent than it is in microbiology or physiology, just two of the biological sciences regarded as basic to medicine. In the face of such complexity, it is not surprising that physicians focus on the practical question of clinical cause. But why, then, do they also speak of cause as if it were simple? The answer seems to be that medicine is a practice, and the ethics of practice, the need to intervene in the patient's illness, works to reduce cause in every case to the simplest manifestation possible. After all, if a proximate cause is known, a treatment can be devised.

Cause—in medicine and out—is seldom simple or linear. Lewis White Beck told a traditional philosophical story to illustrate its complexity.[4] A boy is building a tower of cards. His father sits nearby reading the newspaper; the window is open; the tower grows higher. His mother enters the room; his father puts down his paper; the curtains billow; the boy looks up; the tower falls. What caused the cards to fall? If it were only one thing—for example, if the tower fell every time the door opened—the cause might be watertight. But it looks more complicated than that. The window is open; people are moving. We are free to imagine that if his father had put down his newspaper sooner or (to add complications) if the boy had not been hungrily awaiting his mother's announcement of dinner or if the edge of some particular card had not been a bit irregular, the tower might have stood a little longer. The mother's entering the room or the father's rattling paper may be necessary to occasion the gust or the slight vibration that felled the tower, but as the story stands, these factors are not sufficient. Not only may the tower's collapse have depended on a concatenation of events but the sequence of those events may be crucial.

To admit such contributing circumstances is to tell a story—and for good reason. Narrative captures the subtle, tenuous, vaguely interlocking but clearly temporal relationships among possible secondary or ancillary causes. Neither the card-tower construction nor disease is static. Photography could capture only representative details; video would work better. Events call for narrative representation in time: stories, moving pictures, scenarios, histories, cases.[5] Their contextual details and variation represent tentative hypotheses that, if plausible, might be tested. Experiments could be conducted to establish, for example, the precise relationship among breeze, open window, door, and newspaper. Variables can be controlled. But until the experiments are done, and done conclusively, the interpretive repository of narrative is the most nearly adequate representation of the occurence precisely because of the fertile imprecision of its sequential events unfolding through time. Narrative's causal imprecision and reinterpretability capture and preserve potential causal phenomena in all their possibility.

Illness potentially engages a similar complexity of cause, and biomedical science has done much to pare it down. To questions about how an individual fell ill, germs and viruses and genes—the advances of biomedical science—provide ready answers. The success of the germ theory shaped twentieth-century assumptions about disease causality. Until the late nineteenth century, the largely French and German phenomenological school had argued that disease is a lapse from the physiological norm and restoration of bodily equilibrium is the goal of treatment. English ontologists, somewhat less plausibly, maintained that diseases are objects, invaders to be fought within the body.[6] The discovery of bacteria in the late nineteenth century led to the cure and prevention of many infectious diseases but highjacked the idea of disease causality. With the discovery of the tubercle bacillus, the ontologists seemed to have won hands down. The model of bacterial infection promoted expectations of a linear or mechanistic cause for every disease and a "magic bullet" to cure or prevent each one. It took almost a century of immunology and virology to return to the idea that disease is a physiological disorder: not the necessary but insufficient microbial invader (which in some hosts may produce no effect) but rather the individual's physiological response to it.

What's Going On?

Despite the appeal of a magic bullet, the relationship of cause and effect we attribute to bacteria and viruses is not as linear or conclusive as we might hope. Microorganisms may be necessary to produce infectious disease, but they do not always cause illness. People exposed to a disease can harbor the pathogen—as with tuberculosis or mycoplasma pneumonia—and, though they test positive, still not contract the disease. Why did they not fall ill? And if not everyone exposed becomes ill, why did those who caught the disease catch it? "Why now?"—that quintessentially narrative question—thus becomes important for clinical research and prevention. Those few people, about 5% of the total, who tested positive for HIV antibodies in the 1980s but whose T-cell counts did not fall became the subject of great scientific interest.[7] Something more than exposure, an event beyond the successful introduction of a pathogen into the body, was clearly necessary. The anomaly raised hopes for a clue that would lead to prevention or cure.

Even genes, which seem to offer rock-bottom certainty about disease causality, present a range of contingency. Some genetic mutations, like those for Down's syndrome, are less a cause than a tautological statement of identity: the mutation *is* the disease. With inherited autosomally dominant mutations, the random accident of meiosis and mitosis may appear causal since it is pure chance whether any given child will have one parent's autosomally dominant gene. "Why me?" a person with Huntington's disease could very well ask; "Why me and not my siblings?" Unlike maladies with less than absolute penetrance of the genetic mutation, Huntington's offers no contributory factors that might make a difference. The causal question is clinically uninteresting because it is teleological: beyond prenatal testing and abortion, there is nothing to be done. Other mutations, ones that predispose an individual to disease either by causing the malady or repressing the body's defense against it or both, are causally more interesting. The causal question is recast: "Why now?" Why do only (only!) 85% of women with BRCA mutations develop breast cancer? Why them? Why not the other 15%? Is the disease still to some degree random? The truly interesting possibility for biomedical science is that those 15 in 100 women may not get cancer for some identifiable and replicable reason. The multistep account of cancer etiology—an oncogene that predisposes to cancer and other genes that malfunction so that the cancerous cell is not eliminated—does not answer the question of what sets that system in motion. If a gene does not malfunction from the start, what causes it to malfunction when it does?

To ask this question is to open the question of cause to multiplicative explanation, a move that physicians, despite their preference for linearity, are perfectly willing to make when they must. For breast cancer, sometimes seen as an epidemic with an as-yet-unidentified cause, bodily events and behaviors that increase estrogen exposure have been identified as risk factors: early menarche, late menopause, late pregnancy (or none at all), not breast feeding. Beyond that, a long list of "lifestyle" suspects has been investigated with varying results: alcohol use, dietary fat, pesticides, and other estrogenic chemicals. None of them explains disease in one individual. They are risk factors, not causes, for genetic malfunction.

Despite this complexity of disease causality, a complexity well recognized in medical practice, clinical medicine maintains its far simpler idea of cause. To attribute medicine's simplification of cause to its "scientism" begs the question. Indeed, medicine's most scientific moments occur when clinicians are engaged with the unknown and nonlinear, when a puzzle of diagnosis or treatment bursts its simple causal explanation and compels a more complex, multivariant narrative. This is the recursive interpretation that anomaly provokes, the phenomenon that Richard Rorty, borrowing from Thomas Kuhn, calls "abnormal discourse."[8] "Normal discourse," by contrast, is the unquestioned business-as-usual for which a positivist epistemology works perfectly well. It accounts for the ordinary course of things when effect is seen to match cause and the mechanisms of cause can be assumed as given. Abnormal discourse is provoked when something disrupts this taken-for-grantedness. It resorts to hypothetical narrative, opening the clinical reasoner to new possibilities, new covariants or risk factors.

These creative moments, however, are not medicine's ideal, even though they are highly valued in academic medicine, where they can make a physician's reputation. Even there, the discovery and mastery of complexity enjoy a certain glory only in light of medicine's goal of causal simplicity. Discoveries have no point unless they move medicine toward simplicity in theory and practice. Medicine always works to simplify individual disease causality: the circumstances of the patient's presentation are examined for clues to match the givens of diagnostic etiology until both are absorbed into the obvious: "He had an MI" or "It's lupus." Nothing to it, the implication is. It's cause and effect. Something similar happens with therapy. If a treatment works, it is unlikely to be studied. But new regimens, especially when their side effects are substantial, are pared down in clinical studies until the smallest efficacious dose can be given in the least risky circumstances. Refinements of theory and practice produced by clinical insight and research into complexity may themselves be complex, but their value is tested by their simplifying power in practical use.

Valuing the work of simplification is not the same as regarding the cause of a disease as simple, of course, nor does it require a positivist view of cause. But they seem to help. Why else would medicine ignore the narrative aspect of its enterprise and adopt instead the more rigid assumptions of positivist science? How else could disease—and even illness—seem to fit a two-step, hair-trigger idea of cause and effect? Narratability is the mark of the anomalous in medicine. Settled questions are simple; they scarcely deserve a telling. Narrative, by contrast, is the response to puzzles of diagnosis and treatment, to uncertainty, to the unsolved and problematic. No wonder physicians, who inevitably value normal discourse as a sign of their success, contemn the anecdotal and cling to an idea of science that, however antiquated, promises certainty.

Medicine's simplification of the idea of cause is a consequence of the profession's character as a practice and its goal of acting for the good of the patient, intervening in the course of illness. Normal discourse and the simplification of cause (and with it, it seems, science itself) are the goals toward which it works. Because physicians are committed to act on the patient's behalf and to offer in the process both treatment and explanation, they move to normalize (for themselves as well as the patient) the new phenomena that science produces and the old that escape from a previously satisfactory explanation. Diagnostic reasoning narrows the idea of cause to a single agent, the necessary if perhaps not sufficient sine qua non. Physicians need to pursue the question of cause only well (or long) enough to devise an intervention. If a disease is multifactorial, there is no need to bother with its vexing causality if at least one of its factors is manipulable and can produce an altered effect that will improve or cure the patient's condition. The identification of a cocontributory factor that deters or delays the effects of a disease, like elevated cholesterol or smoking, simplifies the discourse of cause as effectively as an antidote for a malady's necessary bacterial or viral cause does. Robert Aronowitz has described how the discovery of such contributory causes has stripped and scientized wholistic descriptions of maladies not only in poorly understood conditions like fibromyalgia but, more to the point, in readily recognized clinical entities like angina and Lyme disease.[9] Once a causal factor that can be manipulated to alter outcome is identified, discourse is normalized, flattened, simplified. Medicine's interest in the individual's etiology and course of illness is routinized and tends to disappear.

The Misrepresentation of Cause

In the ordinary course of their practice, then, physicians maintain their focus on a simple, linear cause despite recognizing a bewildering array of potential causal factors that they do not (yet) understand and cannot affect. Working to identify the malady or the variable that will enable them to intervene in the course of illness, they translate the patient's story into a narrowly focused medical account and efface themselves as its narrator so as to approximate a scientific objectivity. Multifactorial or multiplicative causality is avoided unless absolutely necessary, which is to say until diagnosis proves difficult or treatment is unsatisfactory. Only then does the idea of cause open, widen. Then the patient's history is reexamined, minutely this time, and the etiology of possible diseases becomes the object of scrutiny. The physician rethinks what is known about pathophysiology or pharmacology, seeks advice, and scours published studies. At such times scientific cause seems the central question in academic medicine. Clinical practice may take scientific cause for granted and prize the normal discourse that focuses on clinical cause, but in university hospitals and tertiary-care medical centers, the discovery of oddities and exceptions becomes the object of professional activity. Their explanation is the coin of academic exchange. Medicine comes to be regarded by its practitioners and by the patients who need their care not as scientific (which it undoubtedly is) but as a science itself.

Physicians are not alone in their need to represent cause as simple. Patients are not much engaged by the multiplicative aspect of cause, and, to judge by the news media, neither is the general public. News reports narrow and flatten the idea as they focus on the research into "the cause" of various life-threatening diseases. There is good reason for this. If the ontologists had been right about more than infectious diseases and the cause, *a* cause, for cancer could be found, then it would be clear how to intervene in the chain of cause and effect that leads to its takeover of the body. Biomedical science would be on the brink of devising a cure. Short of finding a necessary cause, the identification of a contributory cause specifies a point of intervention: remove or alter that secondary cause, and the disease itself will not occur, or its effects will be lessened or eliminated, perhaps repaired. This brilliantly successful approach—especially in the reports of its results—envisions causality as narrowed almost to stimulus and response. And so long as a malady is cured or prevented, who cares! Media interest and the public attention it encourages and reflects do not represent a concern with theoretical knowledge, with science pure and simple, or, even less, with the multileveled character of cause that best represents the understanding of disease. Media interest in biomedical science is, strictly speaking, not a scientific interest at all but a practical concern very like the clinical one. It shares the focus on practical effect, the same focus that drives clinical medicine. When the goal is to ameliorate or eliminate the consequences of disease or injury, almost any cause will do, so long as it can serve as a point of intervention.

Meanwhile, much of clinical discourse in its normal state confirms medicine's idealization of a simple linear causality. When diagnosis, therapy, and prognosis are well established and uncontroversial, the question of cause drops from awareness. If the patient's symptoms are easily recognized and the treatment of choice readily available and not contraindicated in a particular case, there seems to be no science at all. The experienced clinician "just knows."[10] Treatment often then can be reduced to a protocol: a nurse, a physician's assistant, an emergency medical technician, and certainly an intern, perhaps even a medical student, can take over. At such moments—luckily a good part of medical practice—the conventional idea of science seems realized. Physicians understandably identify with such success.

There is more to medicine, however, than its ideal representation or its successes. Illnesses can elude ready diagnosis, and patients may respond in an unexpected way to standard therapy. When a diagnosis cannot be made or treatment is problematic, the case is no longer "normal." It needs redescription, rethinking, analysis. Questions of cause—what is going on here? how is it happening?—become central again. This is why ambulances have radio links to emergency rooms and why interns are supervised. Physicians rethink—renarrativize—the mechanisms of disease; they retrace events in the causal chain or the therapeutic pathway. They go to the library or go online and learn something known to others that they had not known; or they consult with an expert whose work on the problem offers a new way of looking at the case. Sometimes they themselves work out something entirely new about the disease or its therapy, an exception to the known rules that, after confirming research, may become a rule on its own. In this discursive, collective way, clinical knowledge is refined. New diseases are identified; deadly ones inch toward becoming chronic ones; new drugs with unexpected side effects are withdrawn from use.

Medical education has the double task of equipping physicians for the everyday practice of "normal" medicine, when cause is so simplified as to disappear, and for the eruption of the abnormal, when cause becomes a central question, potentially complex and multiplicative. Physicians must keep in mind all that is known to be abnormal in medical practice—like a dementia that could be the now-rare tertiary syphilis or the chest discomfort that is not pain but may signal a heart attack in a 40-year-old woman. They must preserve an awareness that what seems to be an ordinary malady suddenly may be revealed as anomalous. Legionnaire's disease in the late 1970s turned out to be a new type of pneumonia; young gay men with Kaposi's carcinoma, a skin cancer that had been a disease of the elderly, turned out to have AIDS; previously healthy middle-aged people with symptoms of flu suddenly were dangerously ill with SARS.

Physicians preserve this awareness in two ways. They absorb the ideal of medicine as a science, and they rely on the narrative representation of clinical cases. Although identifying phenomena and matching them with diagnoses in the taxonomy of disease resemble the work of naturalists more closely than that of physicists or chemists, the vision of medicine as a science nevertheless fosters an openness to new phenomena and a tentative but progressive, experimental attitude of inquiry. This scientific attitude is reassuring, steadying, even as the work of the clinician often calls for a broader, more circumstantial idea of cause. When an anomaly does appear, the narrative habit, hedged by prohibitions against trusting the single instance, proves invaluable. From the narratological point of view, an anomaly is a narratogenic incident, a disruption of a (till then) unremarkable course of events. The case that reports the oddity is the essential form taken by abnormal discourse in medicine precisely because of narrative's broader, more open and contingent representation of cause. Narrative captures untested causation and lays out hypothetical scenarios that will be discarded or confirmed by experiment. It represents the variables—still imprecise and unstudied—for further investigation. Not surprisingly, then, clinical medicine at its most scientific requires a circumstantial narrative that can describe all the ways the anomalous illness event frustrates established expectations. Despite everyone's best efforts, the malady may remain a fever of unknown origin, an idiopathic disease, or a cancer's metastasis from an unknown primary site. But, more often, with hard work and a little luck, the physician's drive to intervene in the course of the patient's illness will reduce the cause to a simple linearity. The diagnosis of the malady and its treatment, along with its scientific etiology, will become obvious and minimally narratable again, part of the normal discourse of medicine.

The Representation of Clinical Cause

Multiplicative cause and the intractable singularity of the individual case are not news in the social sciences. Through most of the second half of the twentieth century, thinkers in anthropology, sociology, economics, political science, psychology all struggled with the particularity and subjectivity of their knowledge. Historians, especially, had hoped to generalize, even quantify, the purported lessons drawn from past events. But as that retrospective and narrative discipline attempted to construct explanatory models so as to predict the future, it confronted the difficulties inherent in knowing and representing particular experience. The historian Carlo Ginsberg describes the conclusions drawn from that attempt to construct a science from particular events:

> [T]he group of disciplines which we have called evidential and conjectural (medicine included) are totally unrelated to the scientific criteria that can be claimed for the Galilean paradigm. In fact, they are highly qualitative disciplines, in which the object is the study of individual cases, situations, and documents, precisely *because they are individual,* and for this reason get results that have an unsuppressible speculative margin.[11]

Those "evidential and conjectural disciplines (medicine included)" have two ways of representing individual cause when variables are multiple and poorly controlled: statistics and narrative.

While statistics these days needs no apology, narrative needs some justification as a truth-seeking strategy, even in history, that most story-dependent discipline.[12] In fields that cannot—or ethically may not—ignore outliers, narrative is well suited to the representation of singular events, and when those events cannot (or may not) be replicated, retrospective investigation requires narration. Indeed, such representation is almost certainly the reason for its existence. And if it is useful in ordinary, unproblematic situations, it becomes essential when representing (and reasoning about) matters that are circumstantial and uncertain. In the normal discourse of clinical medicine, as I have argued, the "narrative fit" of diagnosis is based in part on scientific data and is likely to be regarded as science—even as that science disappears, absorbed into "just knowing." In abnormal discourse, however, the failure of a standard diagnostic narrative to explain the phenomena of the clinical case is the first clue that something new or not yet understood is going on. In the clinical investigation that will follow, hypothetical narratives play a central role. Restoration of the simplicity of "narrative fit" is the goal first of hypothetical trial and discovery and then of theory selection.

As a part of clinical medicine's narrative rationality, then, the question of cause in clinical practice can be seen as a narrative question and not a scientific one. A larger and much less deterministic sense of cause guides the clinician's interpretive inquiry: What is going on with this patient? Where can medicine intervene? How *should* it intervene, given this patient's life circumstances?[13] Because clinical reasoning is retrospective, it needs to be represented in a way that allows a larger, looser concept of cause than linear cause and effect. What is needed is representation that can accommodate time and chance. Narrative provides for the circumstantiality of (probably) noncontributory detail and leaves room for contingency, conjuncture, and multiplicative causes that unfold over time. This partly random, partly determined concatenation of antecedent events is just what must be controlled in scientific and social-scientific research.

Meanwhile, in clinical medicine, case narrative serves as a repository of events. Written or oral, it not only assembles the history of the patient's illness but also preserves the traces of judgments made, hypotheses eliminated and confirmed, actions taken and discontinued. The case both accommodates the multifactoriality of cause in individual instances of illness and works to normalize events as it records them for later use, including, when necessary, their reinterpretation. If a satisfactory solution is not forthcoming, the case narrative contains details that may prompt a new explanation or a new line of investigation. Thus, clinical narrative serves the goal of diagnosing and treating illness, and all physicians—clinicians, clinical researchers, laboratory scientists—work to simplify every narrative with the hope of reducing it to the bare plot of a readily made diagnosis and an obvious therapy. When they succeed, as they often do, the automaticity, the normality that clinicians value is restored. Chart notes then are brief; oral presentations uninteresting, then forgone. The easy, linear yoking of cause and effect that marks the narrative fit of everyday acts of diagnosis seems to confirm clinical medicine as a successful positivist science.

Thus, despite physicians' focus on the individual case, their backward-facing effect-to-cause rationality, and their reliance on narrative, clinical medicine continues to be described as a science. Its pragmatic and linear causal goal is a part of that claim. Both the claim to be a science and the drive to simplify clinical cause to a bare etiological plot are instruments of a moral enterprise. They grow out of the physician's duty to respond to the needs of ill people, a duty that in the process suppresses curiosity about the credibility or the intellectual status of that claim. Clinicians thus are free to hold sophisticated ideas about the history and philosophy of science and a clear view of the uncertainty of their practice yet simultaneously ignore these insights in favor of their overriding commitment: not to knowledge but to the care of patients.

As a consequence—and in spite of the claim that medicine is itself a science—physicians regularly put the care of the patient ahead of the requirements of science. In their clinical encounters they habitually omit activities that might be expected of a science, including the investigation of the illness's originary cause. What's more, they ignore or circumvent scientific method whenever it is irrelevant or potentially dangerous for the care of the patient. Indeed, guaranteeing this nonscientific focus in clinical medicine is the goal of the Belmont Report on biomedical research and the regulations of institutional review boards that have followed from it.[14] These inconsistencies do not disturb physicians or alter the medical profession's goal of reducing clinical medicine to a set of normal practices or routine protocols based on biomedical science and epidemiology. Far from rendering medicine nonscientific, these oddities shift the profession toward postmodern accounts of knowledge practices in the sciences.

Bruno Latour's account of "hybrids" in *We Have Never Been Modern* contains little about illness or medicine, but his analysis of those contemporary objects of knowledge fits them well. Hybrids, he says, are multidisciplinary social networks of science, politics, industry, social customs, market economics, sexual practices, religion, and governmental policy. Inseparably bound together, they cannot be the exclusive province of any single domain of knowledge. They are "real like nature, narrated like discourse, and collective like society," and they thrive precisely to the degree they ignore the complicated traffic they conduct among nature, discourse, and society.[15] Not only is contemporary biocultural illness a hybrid but the medicine that treats it is an equally complex mix of science, language, and social systems. What's more, medicine's epistemological blindness toward its own complicated way of knowing, in Latour's scheme, is characteristic of a hybrid. Medicine's claim to be a science dealing with nature (or the real) distracts both its practitioners and the rest of us from its disregard of the implications of that claim, even as the profession multiplies its societal and discursive activities. Such duplicity, Latour maintains, is not false consciousness or deception but a failure to connect belief and practice that is essential to a hybrid's function. Medicine's blindness to the incommensurability of its belief and practice—its visual field defect—is, by Latour's lights, necessary for its success. Medicine flourishes precisely because it protects itself from investigation and ignores its narrative and collective aspects. Along with its claim to be a science, medicine's obliviousness to its ways of thinking and working—its epistemological scotoma—enables its actual, covertly nonscientific work of caring for patients as rationally as possible.

The question of cause is central to this conceptual duplicity in medicine. Although clinicians share their reliance on narrative rationality with history, psychology, economics, and the other social sciences, their dedication to finding a cause for the patient's symptoms and their use of biology in that effort seem to support the claim that medicine is a science. Obliviousness to the illogic of this claim and to the oddities of clinical cause enables physicians to identify with the powerful, immensely useful scientific knowledge they draw upon—even as they engage with messy human detail that is poorly controlled, complex, multiplicative, and almost surely impossible or unethical to replicate. Biology and epidemiology are irreplaceably valuable in the care of patients, but medicine's clinical focus is the patient and not the scientific investigation of disease causality. When puzzles arise, medicine's epistemological blindness enables physicians to call un-self-consciously on a richer concept of cause, one that is retrospective, circumstantial, case-driven, narrative. Physicians thus can move easily beyond the simple idea of cause that belongs to medicine's conventional view of science to far more complicated and chancy ideas: necessary but not sufficient variables, covariants, statistical probabilities, risk factors. When anomalies occur, intuitions are tested, cases presented and collected, research stimulated, new information put to use. All the while physicians' practical epistemology—their clinical judgment—and their peculiar uses of the idea of cause are ignored.

Does the misdescription of medicine matter? Perhaps the difference between the profession's aspiration to the status of a science and the way clinicians actually think and work is just an academic distinction, something visible from the outside that makes no difference to the practice of medicine. Physicians, fortunately, do not act on the scientific positivism they revere but continue to reason interpretively, retrospectively, and narratively rather than (as they imagine scientists do) entirely hypothetico-deductively. As long as medicine works, why analyze it? Perhaps this is, as Latour's analysis suggests, the way it must be.

Yet this epistemological blindness, however necessary in the circumstances of practice, involves a costly misrepresentation of the nature of medicine. The misdescription of medicine as a science results in a failure to understand and appreciate medicine's strengths and limits. If the profession were in good health, medical schools were places of real education rather than (all too often) fact-stuffing feedlots, and residency programs were concerned with the character of the clinicians they train, there would be no reason to write a word about it.[16] No one would think to ask the critical interpretive question: What is going on here?

CHAPTER SIX

~~

Clinical Judgment and the Problem of Particularizing

Talk to me
so we can see
what's goin' on . . .

—MARVIN GAYE

IF MEDICINE WERE practiced as if it were a science, even a probabilistic science, my daughter's breast cancer might never have been diagnosed in time. At 28, she was quite literally off the charts, far too young, an unlikely patient who might have eluded the attention of anyone reasoning "scientifically" from general principles to her improbable case. Luckily, medicine is a practice that ignores the requirements of science in favor of patient care.

Deduction is the label Sherlock Holmes uses for his rational skill, and physicians, who find medicine's investigative procedures mirrored in his practice, have adopted the term to describe their thinking. Certainly some of what they do is deduction, but syllogistic reasoning from general rule to particular case is not the particularizing skill that gives them their characteristic strength as clinical thinkers. Anyone in possession of those general rules can apply them to a given case, excluding and confirming the possibilities listed in the differential diagnosis. The construction of that list, however, requires a clinician. Someone well informed, well trained, and experienced is needed to describe the case and decide which rules may apply; only physicians, in other words, can construct the syllogism that the rest of us could work through so easily.

The rule for breast cancer is that firm, well-delineated abnormalities are the cancerous ones and, conversely, other kinds of lumps are usually benign.

If this patient's abnormality is ill defined and feels part of surrounding tissue, then it is probably not cancer. Supplied these facts, the average woman in the street can reach a reliable conclusion. But deduction is only a part of physicians' thinking. How absolute is the rule? Are there lumps that are not firm and well-defined that turn out to be cancerous? (And, less worrisome but still important, are there some firm and well-defined ones that do not?) How accurately has this particular lump been described? When is a nodule or a speck on a mammogram "insufficiently suspicious" and when not? The rule-governed deduction is easy. Doing the work that produces an accurate and reliable syllogism is the difficult part, and so is deciding what to do with its deductive conclusion. Because general rules in clinical medicine are almost never absolute, diagnostic interpretation and decision require clinical judgment. This is what consulting a physician is all about. If the patient with a firm, well-delineated breast mass is 28 years old, and 28-year-olds do not, as a rule, have breast cancer, never mind logic or probability: it needs to be biopsied. If the patient with the suspicious lump is a man, in whom breast cancer is not likely at all and tissue even harder to mammogram, it needs to be biopsied, too. In all these cases, including the obvious, easily deduced one, the clinical skill lies not in the deduction but in what comes before and after: first the detection and the interpretive description of the abnormality, then the construction of the differential diagnosis (fibrocystic disease, fibroadenoma, carcinoma of the breast), and finally weighing the probability of a negative test result against the risk of a positive one.

Clinical judgment, physicians' essential intellectual virtue, is a matter of putting all this together in a balanced way. The pathophysiology of breast abnormalities, which probably does not come to consciousness, underlies the clinical rule; epidemiology establishes the probabilities that govern the order of the differential list; and clinical experience informs physical skill and the awareness of variability. Physicians must know the rules and when to break them, how to use logic and when to ignore its conclusions. Putting it all together, they must decide whether to refer the patient for further tests and with what sort of expectation. The decision is bordered by the possibility of error: the life-threatening mistake of offering statistical reassurance to a man or a 28-year-old woman with a suspicious breast lump; the less serious but still costly error of sending everyone with any sort of mass or mammogram speck for further tests. The act of deduction is logic, and physicians do very well at it: it is neat and satisfying and entirely unremarkable. Their clinical expertise, however, depends on prior interpretation: the ability to understand the particulars of the patient's malady in light of general clinical rules and epidemiological probabilities and to use that body of information to make sense of the patient's symptoms and signs. What characterizes physicians, indeed, in some sense, *makes* them physicians—is their clinical judgment: a more multifaceted interpretive reasoning, including their use of C. S. Peirce's abduction—the logic necessitated by reasoning from effect to cause. They must see the big picture in the particular case, then reason backward to determine whether this patient is an instance of that biological generality, and, finally, know what best to do with all they know or suspect.

Understanding the particulars, despite the inexact relevance of biological science and statistical epidemiology to the circumstances of one person's illness, is medicine's chief moral and intellectual task. In this, medicine differs from biomedical science, which seeks more abstract and generalizable knowledge for a more abstract and general good. Each, of course, needs the other's work to do its own. Biomedicine creates its generalizations from the clinical particulars that are its data, while in turn its conclusions inform and test the work of clinicians, who must use these abstract results to understand the signs and symptoms of the individuals they treat. In calling the subdisciplines of human biology "the basic sciences," physicians imply that biomedical knowledge is both essential and only a part of what they must know. The work of scientists, traditionally understood (and traditionally is how it is understood by physicians), is logically simpler than the practical work of the clinic.[1] Face to face with a patient, physicians must simultaneously call up the potentially relevant clinical and scientific rules and calculate whether those generalizations might apply to this particular ill person. Because even the best scientific and clinical studies are inexactly related to any given individual, even the most knowledgeable and experienced physicians confront the problem of particularization with every patient in every clinical encounter. This is the ineradicable uncertainty of medicine.

Particularization in Clinical Reasoning

Clinical reasoning in medicine has, of necessity, two aspects: generalization and particularization. These are opposite moves—lumping and splitting—and they alternate in tension as the reasoner moves between them. Negotiation between the general and the particular gives clinical medicine its striking intellectual tension. Medicine's counterbalancing movement—or maybe it's a pendulum swing—between the patient's presentation and the established taxonomy of disease is what prompts clinicians to cite exceptions to every rule and then, if needed, to entertain exceptions to those exceptions. This counterweighing is the central characteristic of clinical judgment, the exercise of practical reason needed to reason retrospectively under conditions of uncertainty. Each move—lumping or splitting—serves to test and curb or refine the other.

Generalization, with all its attendant risks, answers the human need to categorize. Practitioners must recognize the phenomena of their discipline. They have to know what's what. Experienced physicians make observations, gather data, test their hypotheses, apply labels, and draw conclusions. New learners recapitulate this process of acquiring and refining knowledge, and clinical researchers extend it. Controlling for variables, statistical studies test observational hunches and common clinical practices. The results are aggregate numbers that can suggest a strong correlation, as the surgeon general's 1964 report on smoking and lung cancer did, or disprove long-held assumptions, like the 1990s Women's Health Initiative study of postmenopausal estrogen use. Such studies correct and advance the necessarily limited case-based experience of even the most expert individual physician.

The other half of clinical knowing is particularization. It is the opposite (or reverse) of generalization, and it is essential to clinical judgment. Faced with a multitude of generalizing studies of varying quality and uncertain relevance, a physician must figure out how any or all of them apply to a particular patient—and, as in cases of patients with a breast lump, decide whether the risks are great enough or the relevance imprecise enough to ignore them. Variables, like age and gender, narrow the quest and, when warranted, prompt further research. Some forms of what seems to be a single disease—lymphoma, for instance, or rheumatoid arthritis—differ enough that treatments and prognoses differ. Researchers ask whether there is some way to shift severe cases toward the mild end of the range, especially now with gene therapy just over the horizon. Occasionally, particularizing research has been prompted by chance. Some HIV-positive patients took unauthorized but at least temporarily successful "vacations" from their medication. Could every patient do the same, physicians wondered, and extend the time the drugs would work? If not, why were these particular people able to? Until focused studies are done, treatment is guided by general research and by clinical experience with its use. If there are no studies that suggest which of the few 28-year-olds without a family history of breast cancer will have malignant breast nodules—"Higher mortality in young women is not completely accounted for by the known prognostic factors"—then clinical practice follows a precautionary rule: biopsy every one.

Both lumping and splitting pose problems. The difficulty associated with generalization, the first half of clinical reasoning, is well understood in medicine. It arises from what seems to be a narrative instinct: human beings construct accounts of cause and effect from whatever evidence is available—

and from apparently random events if they must.[2] Practical reasoners at every stage of expertise can make the mistake, often unconsciously, of generalizing from too few instances or from flawed or insufficient evidence. Rules for reasoning are full of warnings against assuming that what follows an event (post hoc) is therefore caused by it (ergo propter hoc) or that two things appearing together signify a causal relation between them. Likewise, stereotyping—a shortcut in reasoning if there ever was one—is rightly viewed with suspicion: one member of a group cannot stand for every other. In clinical medicine, the error most dreaded is generalizing from a single case, and this is due in part to the anecdote's useful, suggestive power. An anomaly can signal a new response to treatment, a new disease, or a new variant of an old one, but more often it is a deceptive "red herring" that will skew the sense of the whole that the clinician depends on. The well-acknowledged danger of using a single instance as a guide for future practice has made the word "anecdotal" an emblem of all that is unreliable in medicine. But medicine differs from the physical and social sciences, disciplines that may discard oddities and statistical outliers. For physicians the anomalous case is still a patient in need of care. As protective devices, medicine has enlisted logic, "objective" clinical method, and stringent habits of investigation and reportage. Along with the skepticism that underlies them, these correctives often serve as evidence that medicine is a science.

The difficulty with the other half of clinical knowing is less well understood. Particularization is the essential act of clinical reasoning. It begins with the interpretive question that is the focus of every clinical encounter: What is going on with this patient? The inquiry will locate this individual in a general scheme of illness. But as important as particularizing is, it is chronologically and methodologically secondary to generalization. "Lumping" necessarily precedes "splitting." For example, physicians need to know clinical cardiology before they can suspect, much less reliably diagnose, a particular patient's myocardial infarction; statistical studies must exist before anyone can begin to debate how they might apply to a single patient. Yet the particulars, including exceptions to the general rule, remain centrally important. Physicians must know that a very few 28-year-old women really do have breast cancer before they can ignore the studies of its statistical improbability. An understanding of the individual in light of the general is, after all, the clinical point.

A story about a Dublin zookeeper illustrates the medicine's epistemological predicament and suggests why Aristotle declared there could not be a science of individuals.[3] Renowned for breeding lions in captivity, the zookeeper was asked the secret of his success.

"You must understand lions," he said.

"What is it that you have to know about lions?" the interviewer asked.

"Ah, well," replied the zookeeper, "you need to understand: every lion is different."[4]

Evidence-based medicine is designed to address the problem of particularization by enabling physicians to assess clinical research in light of their patients' particular characteristics.[5] How well does a given patient fit the clinical categories that experience and research have constructed? And what should be done when, as often happens, they fit imprecisely or when two diagnostic categories coincide in a single patient? Evidence-based medicine encourages physicians to refine their clinical expertise by searching out and assessing recent studies to answer a well-framed, patient-focused question about some aspect of clinical care: prior probability, signs and symptoms, test results, diagnosis, prognosis, response to treatment, preventive measures, diagnosis, prognosis, or treatment. The first patient in *Evidence Based Medicine* is an overweight 56-year-old smoker with type 2 diabetes and elevated blood pressure. He'd rather stick with the vitamin E and beta-carotene he has been taking for his blood pressure instead of starting antihypertensive medication, and he asks the doctor how the antihypertensive will affect someone who has diabetes. Common sense calls for him to take the medicine despite his diabetes—high blood pressure is serious!—but the evidence-based clinician decides to investigate his question. She finds not only that antihypertensives work just fine for diabetics but that beta-carotene is not recommended for a smoker with high blood pressure.

This is not "cookbook medicine," nor does it replace clinical judgment, two of the charges that EBM has provoked since its introduction.[6] Questions about how large studies apply to an individual patient are extensions of the ordinary work of clinical medicine. The problem of particularization is not hard to grasp; the man with diabetes and high blood pressure certainly understands it. But EBM encounters opposition because clinical judgment and its relation to the problem of particularization are poorly understood. Opponents quite rightly fear—and wrongly see in EBM—a tendency toward generalization without particularization or, to put it another way, a reliance on generalization, one-size-fits-all rule-making, without the particularizing countermove required by clinical judgment and by the ethics of medicine. They fear that the patient with a suspicious breast lump will go untested because as a man the epidemiological evidence is against his having carcinoma of the breast. Or, more realistically, they fear that EBM will be misused: that insurers will not pay for the man's biopsy because it is not statistically indicated. But this is to ignore the work and, especially, the moral obligation of medicine.

Far from promoting wholesale epidemiological solutions to clinical problems, EBM addresses one half of the problem of knowing in an uncertain practice, the problem of particularizing from generalized knowledge. The method can be seen as a contribution to medicine's "phronesiology," the theory of its practical rationality. Because clinical knowing arises from individual cases (however well aggregated in clinical studies) and must ultimately be applied to an individual patient, that knowledge is necessarily circumstantial and radically uncertain. Competent clinicians must simultaneously know the general rules of their practice and recognize exceptions when they occur. They must entertain the possibility of anomalies without letting that possibility distort their judgment. Yet even the best residency followed by a fellowship in the very smallest possible subspecialty cannot provide a physician with an example of every manifestation of disease he or she will need to recognize over a lifetime of practice. People differ, diseases change, new information floods the academic journals. Clinical judgment, when fueled by reliable information and a store of related experience, enables physicians in an unfamiliar situation to work out the best thing, under the circumstances, to do. The methods of EBM do not supply "correct" answers but rather information that can improve clinical judgment. Like the deduction that rules out unlikely diagnoses in the differential list, the answers supplied by EBM depend on the physician's fund of knowledge and experience. Still, clinical judgment is essential for formulating the clinical question and, once obtained, for knowing what to do with the answer in order to care for the patient.

Knowing in clinical medicine requires negotiating both the uncertainties of particularization and the tempting comforts of generalization. Indeed, the two give clinical reasoning its distinctive counterbalancing, tug-of-war character. The need to particularize, one half of medical knowing, exists in tension with the impulse to generalize, and that tension calls for clinical medicine's practical rationality. When one half is asserted, the other is invoked as a challenge. In clinical conferences, the particularizing appeal of clinical experience often goes up against the generalizing authority of "the data," and the two are in constant dialogue (and occasional conflict) in a single clinician's consciousness. Yet this tug-of-war is not static. Like the negotiation between the patient's presenting symptoms and the physician's knowledge of clinical taxonomy, the interaction between the particular and the general homes in on a goal: the diagnosis. Reasoners move abductively from particular to the general and back again, filling out the idea of this patient's malady as they narrow the relevant generalities and test them against the particular details of the case. The opening account of the patient's symptoms matches up with the clinician's knowledge of disease etiology and prompts questions about details that focus the investigation: Anyone sick at home? Any occupational exposure? The answers move the reasoner to a more nuanced consideration of the disease possibilities. Nor does the circle stop here: tests are ordered to refine the description of the patient's malady and (deductively) to confirm suspicions and eliminate false leads. The results, in turn, are interpreted in light of the clinician's store of scientific and clinical information, and, finally, that interpretation is refined by familiarity with this one patient—even sometimes by hunch.[7] A result that would be abnormal in most patients in this instance might be normal; the man with the well-defined breast nodule has women relatives with breast and ovarian cancer. Has that been studied? The good clinician may turn to the database with a well-formed question but schedules a biopsy too.

This abductive, interpretive circle is essential to clinical reasoning. It is the rational procedure necessary in an experiential practice where discoveries, unlike those in biology or physics, must be tested at the same field where they were made.[8] The physician cannot inject a little of the patient's saliva or blood into a volunteer and see what develops.[9] Instead, the history and the physical clues, the symptoms and the signs, must be interpreted as they exist in the patient. They must be understood well enough to point convincingly to a recognizable (or well "lumped") account of disease, and then (in a move to "split") the preliminary diagnosis must return to the patient to be tested against the evidence. From this phronesiological point of view, EBM is the most recent turn of the diagnostic, interpretive circle. To be truly valuable as a refinement in the process of clinical specification, it must prompt new studies of clinical variables in more and more particularized groups of patients—the very research Alvan Feinstein charged that it supplanted.[10]

Not that there can be, scientifically speaking, a study with a sample size of 1—although something very close to that is imagined by the newly conceived gene therapies. For now, that final, singular act of "splitting" eludes science: no study, no matter how carefully matched, can tell a person whether she will be one of the 1 in 10 smokers who contracts lung cancer. Worse, once she falls ill, no study can tell her whether she will be in the small number of patients who will be successfully treated. No matter how fine-grained the research, its results are at most strongly suggestive for an individual. Who can know? Such questions about the individual applicability of generalized knowledge traditionally were settled by clinical intuition, the advice and example of experts, and community standards of care. Uncertainty and imprecision have been tolerated because the ultimate problem of individualization has been insoluble. Yet, as Feinstein suggested, a research focus on clinical phenomena that might take us closer to understanding particular cases is long overdue.

Evidence-based medicine's quest to answer particularizing questions points up the need for such precisely focused studies which can then be mined for their relevance to individual patients. But these clinical studies are not its goal. That goal, like the goal of medicine generally, is how best to take care of a particular patient, given the current state of knowledge. It is medicine's defining ethical and epistemological concern, central to everything else in clinical practice. Evidence-based medicine thus poses the moral questions at the heart of patient care. Given the radical uncertainty of clinical knowing, at what point does a good clinician stop? At what level of generalization? How much investigation into the relationship between the generalizations and the details of this patient's illness is enough?

The Place of the Individual in Clinical Reasoning

Two decades ago, before EBM got its start, a friend from my college years was beginning to play tennis after her third recurrence of breast cancer. She pressed her oncologist, the director of the university cancer center, for a prognosis: How long would this remission last? He told her he didn't know. He had never had a patient so young and athletic and with children still to see through school. There were studies "out there," he said, but who knew how they applied to her?

Could a study be done that would have answered my friend's question? Could an answer be extrapolated from studies that have already been done? Not conclusively, but more could be known. Clinical medicine's focus on the particular does not extend to a concern with or even an interest in establishing a phenomenological account for each instance of disease. Even for an academic oncologist, for example, the causes of a young woman's breast cancer or its recurrence remain all but irrelevant to her diagnosis and treatment. Clinical medicine's duty to act on behalf of the patient subordinates everything else to that overriding concern—including the clinical focus on particular phenomena that may concern her deeply. If the particulars fit the diagnosis and the treatment is well established, that's enough. Physicians have no interest in the individual details or sequences that are not established markers of disease. Nor, despite their empathy, are they interested in the patient's experience of illness. Beyond the clues it supplies for diagnosis, prognosis, and treatment choice, there is no clinical curiosity about individual variation or the history of how this particular patient acquired the disease. Once the clinically relevant details of the case fall into a diagnostic category with no leftovers that demand explanation, there is no further need for investigation. More might be learned, but it would not be useful for the care of this patient. The problem of particularization in this case has been solved.

In the midst of cudgeling my brain about medicine's limited interest in the particulars of the individual case, I stumbled on an illustration of the practical irrelevance of individual phenomena. My new computer came with a game of solitaire, and that game had a replay option. One rainy afternoon, I fell into a brief but virulent fit of repetitive play. As if to justify the waste of time, I discovered that it was a lesson in the elusive relation of cause to effect in the individual instance. Although the rules of the game were inviolable—no cheating, of course, and no peeking either—the replay option meant I could begin the game again whenever I was stuck. Cards reappeared on the screen, laid out exactly as they had been five minutes earlier. Hindsight became foreknowledge in a way not usually found in the real, unreplayable world, and once armed with experience I had a chance to avoid the moves that had blocked my success. I could play every useful card I turned up or hold them back to use with others I now knew were in the deck; I could move the seven of clubs instead of the seven of spades. I could pile cards on the freed aces or leave them in place and draw off lower cards that earlier had left me floundering in an unyielding round of three-card deals. Sometimes replaying a hand worked: the third or fourth time through, a card that had been hidden would turn up and free cards that had been frozen before. I'd win.

Other times, no matter how I replayed it, winning remained impossible. Once an essential red eight was stuck near the bottom of a pile, and the black seven on the top couldn't be moved without a red eight. Several times, overconfident or too focused on a new plan, I'd realize I'd left a moveable card in place for several three-card deals. Had I missed something vital? Never, no matter how I focused, were the replayed games exactly alike. Still, my control of the outcome grew: information increased, practical theory-making burgeoned, and my score improved.[11] At a macro level, the games were the same: the positions of the cards were a given, unchangeable fact that set the limits and perhaps the character of each game. But within those limits, events were minutely variable. Like the time-traveler's footsteps away from the path in Ray Bradbury's story "The Sound of Thunder," a move that alters world history eons later, they had an interconditional contingency.[12] The events of each game—and thus the game itself and its outcome—were more or less different each time. The question of cause in each case was multiplicative, and as a result each game was to some degree uncertain.

And here's the interesting thing: a particular outcome might be reached by several paths. There were many ways to lose, of course, and occasionally (I felt sure) there was only one sequence of moves that would lead to winning. But sometimes I could uncover all the cards in more than one way. Even more specific outcomes—like the number of cards piled on the aces or, most particular of all, the number and identity of those cards (say, the two of clubs, the three of diamonds, the three of hearts, and the five of spades)—could also be achieved by more than one path. There were always sequences of events that produced a given result and sequences that would not, but for most games there was not just one sequence of events necessary for a specified outcome. Were I to reconstruct the means by which a particular result came about, much could be learned and a theory of retrospective determination no doubt could be generated, perhaps even some rules of play. But such rule-governed play could not guarantee that the outcome could be replicated. Nothing but keeping an exact record of moves made and following it precisely a second time could do that, and even then it might not be the only way to achieve that outcome. As historians and other social scientists know well, this degree of replicability is possible only because a 52-card game with inviolable rules is a very small world.

Certainly solitaire is a very much smaller universe than biomedicine. Scientists have the advantage of reducing the range of their inquiry to something small enough to be well controlled. Clinical medicine can often approximate this strategy: blood and urine are tested; x-rays and scans are done. The results, especially in combination, are useful, often conclusive. Sometimes physicians are accused of thinking reductively about patients and of seeing them only as malfunctioning body parts. They are attempting to control the variables in the thought experiment that constitutes diagnosis. This reductive method is useful for narrowing a problem so that it can be posed syllogistically and enable them to confirm or rule out diagnostic possibilities. But, like deduction itself, the method is a part of the conventional, positivist conception of cause that by itself is inadequate for the care of patients. Biological science can establish the character and limits of a physical state, but how the variables play out for a particular human being in a given time and circumstance is largely unknown. Events, even foreseeable ones—their order and timing and therefore their importance—are contingent. Although they will have a pattern, and in some imaginary microcalculable sense they are determined, they cannot be precisely, absolutely predicted. They can be studied statistically in the aggregate, but individually they are known only in retrospect, historically. Establishing the chain of causality for a particular patient's illness or predicting its outcome is thus far more like a replayable solitaire game than the controlled and simple linear process physicians associate with a positivist concept of science. When faced with new instances of what we recognize as "the same thing," even if we are informed with reliable probability studies, we nevertheless cannot be sure what will happen next. Statistics narrow the range, providing very good guesses. But who knows? This time the card we most need may stay hidden.

For all the reasons my solitaire game suggested, physicians have a limited interest in individual causality. However useful in supplying clues for diagnosis, the events that contribute to a patient's illness—its genesis, the course it takes, the effects of treatment, its prognosis—are environmental, circumstantial, more-than-biological matters that are difficult to pin down precisely because they are ungeneralizable, interdependent, microhistorical questions about an individual. The presence of bacteria or an environmental toxin or a genetic mutation may be the necessary cause, but that alone is often not enough to bring on the actual illness. What else happened? Circumstances must be right. Studying these contextual, contributory factors can lead to the discovery of ways to avoid a recurrence or an exacerbation of the disease in a patient who is already ill or to prevent the same disease in other people. Other times, potential contributory factors—like my friend's return to avid tennis playing—are so resistant to experimental control as to be all but useless to both investigator and clinician.

In the clinical encounter, then, epidemiology joins biomedicine not as an answer but as a given set of information to be interpreted and applied to a particular patient. The strategies of evidence-based medicine can focus that interpretation and help narrow its application to an individual. Together these stores of information and the means of mining them are the best we currently know about the way the cards are dealt. Physicians still must turn the cards over, move them empirically, make decisions about strategy, theorizing about *this* case, even, if necessary, playing their hunches. The single case, even when everything is known about it that can be known, must always be viewed comparatively, historically, narratively.

Probabilities, Risk Factors, and Individual Cause

Physicians' practical stance toward the question of cause in the individual case, not surprisingly, becomes a settled attitude that makes it difficult to interest them in statistics or in preventive measures for maladies that may not befall a given patient. The concept of individual cause is valuable primarily for the clues it supplies for diagnosis. Occupational exposures, family history, recent travel, and what in the HIV era have been labeled "risk behaviors"— intravenous drug use and unprotected, especially anal, sex—suggest disease possibilities and render the results of tests for those possibilities more accurate and reliable for that individual.[13]

The same details also guide prevention, a prospective, more hypothetical use of individual phenomena than diagnosis. Here individual causality is invoked for effects that have not yet occurred. Aspects of the patient's life are identified that, if altered, might reduce the likelihood of disease in the future. Like biological cause, epidemiological probability makes persuasive rhetoric when physicians attempt to change their patients' behavior. Start exercising, clinicians will advise; lose weight. Stop smoking; use condoms and clean needles. These cautions draw upon well-established risk factors common to many instances of the malady in question. They are good bets, but how they apply to any given patient is still a guess. Even relatively sure things, like the connection between smoking and lung cancer, are aggregate correlations and do not necessarily apply to this particular smoker. After all, 9 out of 10 smokers will not contract lung cancer—if only because many die of cardiovascular disease or emphysema instead. Secondary prevention, preventing the recurrence or exacerbation of a disease, also evokes individual causation. Avoid the barracuda steak next time, the physician will advise, even though many barracudas are free of neurotoxins. Lose weight and you will probably eliminate what is probably sleep apnea, the firm diagnosis of which would require extensive (and expensive) neurological tests. This prospective reasoning is based on what is known about the statistically established contributory causes of conditions like this patient's. However well-studied the cause, the effect in any given case remains at best a good precautionary guess.

Such patient-focused preventive measures have had a mixed success in the United States, where first fee-for-service payment and then time limits imposed by managed care have worked against them. But the habits of clinical thinking pose an obstacle, too. Prevention has been most successful where "risk factors," those statistically possible contributory causes, have been reframed as diseases or, at the very least, treatable clinical conditions. Elevated blood pressure, high cholesterol, obesity, and smoking, all more or less important in contributing to a given disease, are seldom necessary causes and never sufficient ones. Biological and epidemiological research establishes their force, but the question of their relevance for the individual cannot be answered conclusively. Risk factors, nevertheless, have gained a place in clinical medicine simply because physicians can do something for them. As Robert Aronowitz describes it, preventive measures have been smuggled into clinical medicine disguised as treatment for quasi-diseases such as hypertension and elevated cholesterol.[14] The frame has been changed from solving hypothetical problems that may never occur to addressing practical clinical problems—reducing cholesterol, lowering blood pressure—in the here and now. These risk factors differ from phenomena-like elevated insulin levels because they are predictors rather than signs of present disease; yet they engage the physician's need to do something, to act for the good of the patient.

Along with adjuvant chemotherapy, this preventive treatment of the statistics comes as close to therapy by numbers as medicine gets. Rather than intervening in a retrospective narrative diagnosis, one chosen from a list of likely diseases according to the specificity of the patient's symptoms, the physician's treatment of risk factors aims at forestalling a hypothetical narrative that has yet to unfold. The precise role of risk factors, especially for an individual patient, remains a complex question. Experimentation in this one patient is impossible. Successful treatment of probabilities can be judged only epidemiologically, in the aggregate, not by the alteration it is presumed to make in any given patient's life. Meanwhile, however, the cholesterol level has gone down, and so has the risk of a heart attack. The ex-smoker has lowered her risk of lung cancer and has given up hormone replacement therapy because it turned out to increase, not lessen, the risk of heart disease.

This use of statistical clinical research to treat clinical conditions that foreshadow life-threatening disease does not alter the practice of medicine. It does not challenge the accommodations clinical medicine has made with the problem of particularizing or physicians' practical lack of interest in pursuing details of individual cause. Indeed, it may extend practice as usual. Reframing "risk factors" as clinically treatable diseases calls on medicine's simplest, most generalizing causal patterns and restores uncertainty to its usual manageable position. Here in the present is a treatable condition only a little more uncertain than the rest. It fits easily with the problem of particularization that makes the whole enterprise of clinical medicine radically uncertain. The future no longer stretches into unpredictability; prognosis returns to its customary level of uncertainty. The clinician's reluctance to engage individual phenomena that are "clinically irrelevant"—either useless for diagnosis or untreatable—is left in place.

That reluctance makes good sense. First, there is the sheer logical difficulty of reaching a reliable conclusion about cause in a particular instance of disease. The idea of cause is notoriously slippery in an individual case when reasoning prospectively from cause to effect, the way scientists are believed to do. Second, obtaining conclusive proof is likely to pose ethical problems. Prospective experimentation, which is the scientific way to nail down cause-to-effect hypotheses, has led to the great scandals of clinical research: the injection of retarded children with hepatitis at Willowbrook and the passive observation at Tuskegee of the progression of syphilis in a group of affected black men even after a cure was found. Above all, establishing the individual etiology of a patient's disease is not compelling in clinical medicine because, beyond the diagnostic usefulness of the history of the illness, the steps by which one individual fell ill at a particular time are too multifactorial to be usefully addressed. Besides, it is too late. The phenomena are lost to investigation; the patient is already sick. Medicine does not engage those contributory factors it cannot alter. As a colleague of mine once remarked, "Nothing is a fact unless it's relevant to patient care." Only when the diagnosis is difficult, a treatment unexpectedly fails, or a new disease like HIV or SARS emerges is the question of individual cause opened. Otherwise, pursuing the question of what caused this one individual's illness seems perilously close to teleology: *why* did this person fall ill? About Aristotle's final cause, biomedical science and clinical epidemiology have nothing to say.

Teleology and Individual Cause

For patients, however, the question of individual causality looms large. Why me? Why now? Did I eat too much fat, overdose on saccharin or coffee or preservatives? Did I live too near a toxic waste site, an asbestos plant? The hope of regaining control is buried in these questions. The impersonality of scientific cause and the randomness it often implies—"it just happens"—is bleak and unmalleable. For a suffering individual, the random injustice of the universe has little appeal.[15] If causal agents can be identified, we feel the illness event could have been otherwise. Cure and restoration might still be possible. In the absence of answers—and sometimes in their presence—patients turn to Aristotle's final cause: not How? but the teleological Why? What is the ultimate reason for such an unbearable, unthinkable thing as illness? Especially for those with life-defining conditions, thinking about risks and predispositions readily moves toward larger, even more imponderable questions of meaning. "How is it possible?" becomes "Why has this happened?" especially when treatment choices are evenly weighted or the prognosis a matter of grim statistics. This is neither the scientific question of cause nor a question of what has caused one particular individual out of all others to fall ill but a question of ultimate purpose, a final cause. As Grace Gredys Harris discovered in both Kenya and western New York, sick people give moral reasons for their condition—guilt, anger, and disordered, toxic human relations.[16] Desperate to restore some order to the world, human beings seem entirely willing for that order to be a punitive one. However terrifying, personal agency offers hope that the whole thing may be undone and control regained.

Patients often bring these teleological questions to physicians. In a secular culture, physicians are more conversant with last things than many of the rest of us. Treatment, prognosis, prevention, the management of chronic illness all raise practical clinical questions that are a hair's breadth from the overriding existential one: How should we live the limited life we have before us? Yet physicians' interest (as physicians) in individual causality is constrained by the logical limitations of their retrospective method and by their belief that medicine is a science. Despite their patients' need, such questions may make physicians uneasy. Neither science nor medical education addresses the problem of final cause. Intellectualizing patients readily translate the teleological questions—Why has this happened?—into the puzzle of individual causality: How has this happened? Not surprisingly, physicians are likely to make the same substitution, and it is a flight to the safely tautological. Once the patient's diagnosis is established, the illness seems simply an expression of its etiology in the individual. The patient's malady becomes a particular instance of that disease's general rule, and thus the problem of individual causality is rendered unremarkable. The physician is safe: the fit between disease etiology and causal factors found in the patient's history stands as proof of the diagnosis. This neatly circular identification of the patient's symptoms as instances of a general rule manifesting itself in a particular patient reinforces the sense that medicine is, after all, a science. On scientific grounds, the teleological question—and an awareness of the patient's suffering that lies behind it—can be set aside or ignored.

But physicians are not scientists. They have a different responsibility, and their honesty about medicine's uncertainty can contribute to their care of the patient. If the teleological question is posed directly or if they can hear the question as it is indirectly asked, physicians are in a unique position to address the problem of individual cause in a nonjudgmental, even a healing way. While their use of statistics reinforces their practical certainty, they nevertheless cannot be sure how a patient became ill at this point in life. Faced with a smoker soon to die of lung cancer, they cannot say why other smokers are still disease-free. They cannot even say that if the patient had not smoked, he would not have contracted lung cancer. Statistical research and the metastudies of the Cochrane Collaboration that reconcile (as far as possible) disparate studies have increased the reliability of explanatory and predictive statements, but the reassuring concreteness of numbers cannot leap to the ultimate act of particularization. Physicians do not know why disease exists. No one does. And while they know a lot about patients' diseases, one of the things they know best is that every one of them is different.

PART III

The Formation of Clinical Judgment

CHAPTER SEVEN

⌐⌐

Aphorisms, Maxims, and Old Saws:
Some Rules of Clinical Reasoning

Every physician is a different kind of gambler.

—ERNEST W. SAWARD

CLINICAL JUDGMENT IS not a skill separable from a well-stocked fund of sci-entific and practical information.[1] To provide good care to their patients, physicians must know human biology—both normal and pathological. Yet if science were all that physicians needed, patients would be able to consult a user-friendly computer program and never need to see a doctor at all. Some-times it seems as if medicine is already halfway there, especially when expert panels create algorithms that map successive decision points in a patient's diagnosis or treatment. (See, for example, one of the National Comprehensive Cancer Network's Practice Guidelines in Oncology, Figure 7-1.)[2]

Helpful as these diagrams of decision pathways are, clinical reasoning is far more situated and flexible than even the most complex clinical algorithm can express. These decision trees are aids to clinical judgment—teaching the young and reminding the old—but they are not a substitute. While the tension inherent in medical decision-making is regularly resolved, it regularly reappears. Medical schools and residency programs must cultivate a capacity for complex and flexible but often inconclusive clinical reasoning. The learners, luckily, are intelligent, but they are also (most of them) longtime students of science who are not used to negotiating ambiguous alternatives or to tolerating incomplete or uncertain answers. The solution is not more book-learning but experience: years of clinical apprenticeship spent taking care of patients and steadily reviewing cases and the reasoning that has gone into their diagnosis and treatment. To reinforce these case-based lessons, learners are encouraged to think of the work of diagnosis and treatment as science and at the same time to improve their clinical judgment in ways that ignore or subvert that claim. This contradiction is reflected in informal rules of clinical reasoning that make perfect sense one by one but, taken together, seem to cancel each other out.

Chief among these contradictory rules are the old saws, adages, and aphorisms that concern the clinical encounter. They embody the practical wisdom of experienced clinicians, and almost every one of them can be opposed by another maxim, rule of thumb, or old saw of equal weight and counterforce. For example, Occam's razor, the rule of parsimony, exists side by side with the reminder that people who are old or poor sometimes have more than one undiagnosed disease. No one regards this as contradictory, partly because no one thinks about these maxims much at all. They express the complex relation of knowledge and action in a field where information changes, its application is circumstantial, and, as clinicians often say, "Nothing is ever one hundred percent." Although the existence and value of these maxims now and then have been noted, they have not been studied.[3] As a summary of experience, they have an authority very different from test results and statistical studies. Far more ad hoc and personal, they can be challenged but are not precisely testable. Individual clinical teachers may polish their favorites, consider whether they have repeated them too often, even whether to utter them at all. But no one in academic medicine convenes a teaching conference on the pedagogical use of maxims and aphorisms; nor does anyone—teacher or learner—seem to be troubled by the fact that one may conflict with another. As part of the currency of medical discourse, this colloquial wisdom passes all but unnoticed, part of the tension inherent in the clinical judgment it guides and represents.

Despite this low profile, clinical maxims play an important role in the case-based interpretive process that characterizes knowing in clinical medicine. They guide the development and exercise of clinical judgment, and they model the way it works in practice. In academic medical centers, these informal rules are a tacit part of the ongoing case-based inquiry into the relation of knowledge and action in the care of particular patients, an inquiry that takes place daily, almost hourly, on every specialty service. Discussions of individual cases—narrative accounts of medical attention beginning with the patient's presentation of symptoms—embody the clinical reasoning that is the goal of medical education. They replicate the thought process engaged by every physician, in and out of academic medicine, silently or with colleagues. In conversation, these case discussions constitute much of the collegiality

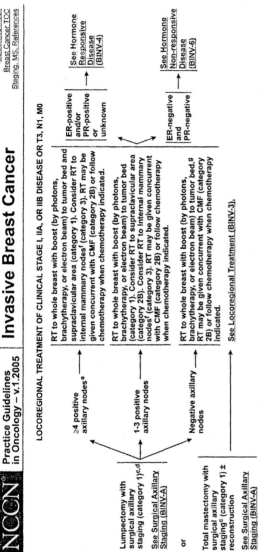

FIGURE 7-1. Reproduced with the permission of NCCN

in medicine. In conferences, case presentations are the pedagogical tool for scrutinizing the rational steps of diagnosis and choice of treatment. In this way, cases are the focus of rituals that educate students and residents and maintain the skills of experienced clinicians. On such occasions, senior physicians reflecting on a troublesome case will utter an aphorism or allude to a familiar maxim: "At this point," an attending physician might say, "I'd let go of Occam's razor." The sayings have the ring of communal wisdom; they counsel the young and often trump the opposition. As a reminder of the weight of accumulated experience, they can be an effective means of closing a discussion or turning it in a new direction. They are medicine's summary guidelines, the rules of thumb for clinical reasoning.

Aphorisms and maxims guide the acts of practical reasoning essential to patient care: history-taking, the physical examination, diagnostic reasoning, and therapeutic choice. They offer provisional rules for the decisions vital to the quality of that care. Not that they are definitive or absolute. Far from it. Alone, clinical maxims can reek of certainty, especially when uttered by a senior physician. But every one of them is qualified or contradicted by another maxim delivered with equal authority or by that maxim's clear disregard in practice. The sayings thus fall into an inherently skeptical, counterweighted pattern of contradictory pairs. In this they resemble proverbs more generally: "A penny saved is a penny earned," but "You can't take it with you"; "Silence is golden," although "Honesty is the best policy." Such contradictory advice is possible, even necessary, because maxims and aphorisms are practical, situational guides rather than invariant axioms or laws. In medicine, each maxim in a counterweighted pair aims for a judiciously balanced application of generalized scientific or clinical knowledge to an individual patient. Once the clinician chooses to follow one—and it is impossible to follow both at once—it is as if the opposite maxim sinks from view. Indeed, clinicians are no more likely to think of these aphorisms as paired and contradictory than the rest of us are to see nonclinical proverbs that way.

Taken as a whole, medicine's paired and counterweighted aphoristic wisdom suggests that while there are clearly wrong answers in the care of patients, there is often no invariably right one. They reveal that clinical education—the demonstration and transmission of clinical judgment—is in part a tug-of-war between competing admonitions about the best course of action. Medicine could be practiced and learned without these old standbys, but their wide and regular use is a reminder that, while physicians work toward certainty, they must act in its absence. Maxims, aphorisms, and old sayings impart situational wisdom, but, even more important, they model situational, case-based practical reasoning.

History-Taking

"The diagnosis is usually made from the history."

"The patient denies alcohol use."

One of the most venerable pieces of clinical wisdom concerns the patient's account of the illness. "Listen to your patient," young physicians are traditionally counseled. "He is telling you the diagnosis." This is often stated as a statistical rule that asserts an approximate probability: "80% [in some versions 90%, but always at least three-quarters] of your patients can be diagnosed from the history."[4] But this wisdom, however strongly stated or well confirmed by thinkers in medical informatics,[5] has uphill work to do against medicine's ingrained skepticism about the history, history-taking, and, especially, the patient as a reliable historian.

Clinical skepticism is clearest in accounts (written or oral) of the patient's presenting narrative. "The patient denies any history of alcohol use, IV drug use, or risk factors for HIV," a medical resident will declare in the conventional language of case presentation—even when the patient is an 82-year-old great-grandmother with no symptom or life circumstance suggestive of such a history. She's the widow of a clergyman as well? It makes no difference. Everyone has had a case like *that*—or has heard of one.

Professionalized doubt about the reliability of sources is shared by all recorders of history. Physicians are especially dependent on the personal report of events by the individual most affected, and, like political and social historians, they are well aware that the information they gather, even from a well-intentioned, honest informant, is always narrow, incomplete, and potentially flawed. Like those historians and the biographers who are their near relations, physicians must be as sure as possible of their data even if, unavoidably, they exercise creativity in putting together the information they elicit.[6] For this reason, the patient's account by custom is labeled "subjective," although, as critics like William Donnelly point out, it is no more subjective than the physician's observation of the clinical signs.[7] This skepticism does not erase the value of the patient's story. The physician's article of faith, that the patient "knows" the diagnosis or its pathognomonic clues and is by far the most important source of diagnostic information, is not inconsistent with an all-purpose skepticism: the belief that truth is less "out there" to be discovered than constructed by the clinical observer. Yet over time, in the community of discourse that is clinical medicine, that larger epistemological skepticism gives way to a persistent, commonsensical suspicion of the patient's reliability and an unwillingness to waste time, look foolish, be misled, or, worst of all, be duped.

The value of the history remains, even as a head CT scan is ordered before a routine lumbar puncture can be performed on a fevered patient with a supple neck and no hint of headache. After all, 5% or 15% or perhaps even 25% of patients *cannot* be diagnosed from their history, and this patient may be one of them. Besides, in the care of patients, a potential exception with an irreversibly bad outcome outweighs statistical probability. Two or three emergency room patients with no signs of increased intracranial pressure reportedly have died from lumbar punctures? Better get a head CT on this one. Thus, contradictory beliefs about the reliability of the patient's history have come to coexist side by side. So long as the risk to the patient is minimal, each serves as a corrective to the other.

"Always record the chief complaint in the patient's own words."

"If he says he has 'gallbladder trouble' . . . ignore it."[8]

Attitudes toward the patient's chief concern epitomize the tension about the reliability of the patient's history. At least as early as the creation of the Atchley-Loeb interview form in the 1920s (still in use at Columbia University), students were asked to record the patient's answer to the opening clinical question, "What brings you here today?" in the patient's own words.[9] Yet long under suspicion, the "chief complaint" (CC) or "presenting complaint" is sometimes viewed as all but useless in this medically sophisticated time.[10]

Despised and undercut, the patient's presenting concern nevertheless can be found in the case write-ups of almost every academic medical institution, although seldom these days recorded in the patient's own words. "CC," the chart might record: "s.o.b." Shortness of breath is resolutely *not* a diagnosis although good clinical procedure forbids jumping to a diagnostic conclusion no matter how obvious—even if the patient literally reports it.[11] "S.o.b." is an intermediate construction, a medicalized symptom, the physician's interpretation as history-writer. Few people come in saying, "I'm short of breath." Instead, they say, "I've been having trouble breathing" or "I can't seem to pull the stairs like I used to," with a dominant hand high and flat on their chest. Are the words "shortness of breath" always an accurate medical translation? And how many of the few patients who actually say the words are short of breath in just the way the physician understands it as he or she writes, a little too easily, "s.o.b."? George Engel, throughout his teaching career, regularly demonstrated the clinical peril of too quickly interpreting the patient's account as fact: "spitting up blood," he liked to point out, is not "coughing up blood."[12] In *Talking with Patients*, Eric J. Cassell argues that recording the patient's own words is "valueless" unless the clinician takes a good history so those words can be understood. He believes, too, that the chief complaint must be addressed before the clinical encounter is over. Does the patient sleep in a sitting position? Need help with daily activities? or with those stairs? It is all the more important, he says, if the presenting complaint turns out not to be the medical problem—and especially if there is no "objective" medical problem at all. [13] Unlike the history as a whole, which is both unanimously revered and universally suspect, there is no consensus on the value of the chief complaint. The patient's words may mislead or they may provide an important clue—or both. Learners will hear a maxim on either side of the question.

Preliminary Hypotheses

> "Always do a review of systems."

> "A good clinician has an index of suspicion . . ."

In the initial interview with a patient, should the physician's mind be a blank slate? Or is it an intuitive steel trap ready to close upon the first good hint? Traditionally medical students are cautioned against a premature narrowing of the diagnostic focus. To reinforce this they are taught always to do a review of systems, in which—no matter how specific the chief complaint or how well it is supported by the patient's medical history—they ask questions about the other organ systems of the body. [14] Like the custom of recording the chief complaint and other symptoms as subjectively reported bodily facts rather than starting off with a diagnostic label, the review of systems is part of the suspension of diagnosis held to be essential to clinical objectivity. This survey of the rest of the body is a pledge of the physician's refusal to jump to conclusions, a hallmark of clinical thoroughness, the antidote to premature (and thus often inadequate) diagnostic closure. "Any chest pain? Any change in bowel habits?" "How is your hearing?"

Yet most physicians can tell stories of diagnoses that they or their illustrious professors "nailed at forty feet." "I walked into the room and I could tell right away—," a physician will say. Whether from the history or the patient's appearance, "every good clinician has an index of suspicion, a clinical intuition . . ." another explains. A chief of dermatology, six months after the event he describes, still sounds amazed: "I hadn't seen a case since I was in the air force in Biloxi twenty years ago, fresh out of residency. But the minute she walked in, the signs were unmistakable. I did a history, of course, but I knew what it was the whole time."

Only relatively recently has there begun to be a serious consideration of the concept of clinical intuition.[15] Leaps of diagnostic insight involve the skillful reading of signs, many of which—like clubbing of the finger ends—are well established in clinical lore. Like the feats of Sherlock Holmes, some skillful reading by expert clinicians is so rapid or "compiled" as to be all but unde-tectable.[16] Such leaps use subtle (or less often taught) social signs. Faith Fitzger-ald has enumerated many of these: the evidence of clothing, body habitus, and possessions on the nightstand.[17] She brings to consciousness the often un-acknowledged details that inform the experienced observer: lopsidedly worn shoes, chipped fingernail polish, asymmetric holes in a recently let-out belt, an untanned strip on the left ring finger. Beyond this clinical semiotics, Patricia Benner, a pioneer in describing the relation of intuition to the development of clinical expertise, has argued that experts actually forget the rules of diagnostic procedure and orient themselves situationally with each new patient.[18]

With research into clinical reasoning and the diagnostic process, the relation between clinical intuition and the review of systems has become clearer. Given that a fund of information relevant to the case at hand is essential to clinical judgment, the review of systems is an intelligent fallback strategy for those who are either not yet (or not in this instance) experts. When Jerome Kassirer and G. Anthony Gorry looked at the self-reported reasoning processes of ex-perienced clinicians presented with the case of a patient suffering from kidney failure, they discovered that nephrologists, the appropriate specialists, asked relatively few questions in order to reach the diagnosis, while equally expert cardiologists, in this case out of their field, resorted to a review of systems. "Headaches?" they asked. "What did you take for them?" "How many?" "Every day? For how long?" Although they asked many more questions than the nephrologists, the nonexperts were able to reach an accurate diagnosis: analgesic-induced kidney failure.[19] Given a good stock of general clinical knowledge, a physician's survey of apparently unrelated organ systems proves invaluable in the absence of the specific, detailed information and specialized experience that constitute expertise. The habit of conducting a review of systems with every patient, inculcated early, remains the default mode for clinicians who are not in the grip of an overriding, fully satisfactory hunch.

Progress in understanding diagnostic reasoning has recently led to the modification of teaching strategy. Rather than being given a procedural rule that will be contradicted by the expert practice they observe with their clinical instructors, some students are now advised to proceed as those elders do, by forming a general idea of the malady—a "working diagnosis"—early in the clinical encounter, then testing and refining it as the interview and examination proceed.[20] It will be interesting to see whether this practical acknowledgment of the way diagnostic reasoning really works will be as successful as the traditional use of contradictory instructions. Will these new physicians be as thorough? Or will they be too confident of their first impressions? Will they resort to a review of systems at the right moment? Or, lacking the injunction to "always do a review of systems," will they stick with a narrowed vision too long or miss comorbidity, a second disease? This new method abolishes the old contradiction that counseled physicians both to suspend judgment and to form an initial impression of the diagnosis. As it diminishes the traditional tension between those competing demands, it no doubt reduces the corresponding tension in the student's psyche. But it risks eliminating what was valuable in the old contradiction: its insurance for beginner and routinized practitioner alike of a certain balance, a consciousness that, no matter which way they may work through a diagnosis, there is another way of proceeding.

Physical Examination

> "Fit clinical observations to known patterns."

> "Take account of every detail and weigh them all carefully."

Like the medical history, the physical examination poses the question of whether the clinician should focus on the immediately apparent malady or the full spectrum of bodily signs and symptoms. Students learning the procedures of the physical examination are advised to pursue their clinical suspicions.[21] At the same time, they are warned not to ignore or fail to give proper weight to any single finding. It boils down to "Focus!" and "Notice everything!" Each, of course, is good advice. The maxim "Fit clinical observations to known patterns" counsels reasoners to work by means of medicine's well-established taxonomy: the pattern for heart disease, for example, may also involve impaired lung function. This is practical help in threading the thicket of clinical signs. After all, as Perri Klass observed in a moment of witty despair, "all written descriptions of all clinical presentations of all diseases are similar: if you list every possible presenting symptom, eventually they all overlap."[22] But what if, in the process of fitting shortness of breath to the pattern of congestive heart failure, the clinical student fails to notice lung disease? The second rule applies: notice everything, take it all into account.

What do judicious physicians do with what they have noticed when a detail does not fit a standard pattern? And what happens when a thorough investigation, meant to be confirmatory, turns up an anomalous sign? Often it is just that ill-fitting detail—hearing an inspiratory rub that does not sound like the "ordinary" pleural rub or a noticing a splinter hemorrhage in a fingernail—that leads to a more precise diagnosis or to a more efficacious treatment.[23] But an ill-fitting detail, especially well into an investigation, is just as likely to be a red herring.[24] A physician must be thorough. And efficient. Thus, when a younger physician, puzzling over an ominous but ill-fitting test result, stands poised on the brink of a "cascade of uncertainty,"[25] preparing to order more complicated, expensive, more invasive tests to determine the reason for the unexpected lab value, wise clinicians—the very people who earlier may have urged careful weighing of all the data—are likely to advise, "Stick to your guns. The lab could have made a mistake. Do the test again."

Tests

> "The best medicine is to do as much nothing as possible."[26]
>
> Sutton's law

Maxims also express the clinical tension between watchful waiting and the "full court press." Because the testing options are so numerous as to constitute whole layers, new algorithms, in the process of clinical reasoning, physicians must be as knowledgeable about the options and the dangers, benefits, and limitations of available tests as they are about the treatment that positive test results will entail. Good clinical practice includes the ability to choose tests wisely and in the most efficient order so as to minimize pain, blood draws, financial cost, and time elapsed till diagnosis. Often these goals conflict, and so, therefore, does the received wisdom about testing strategy. The ideal, of course, is the diagnosis that can be made with certainty from a pathognomonic sign or symptom: a pain like an elephant sitting on a middle-aged man's chest, yellow eyeballs, or a tender, swollen temporal artery. Next best is the single, sensitive, specific, wholly reliable test.

But many diagnoses are not so easily made. Law XIII in Samuel Shem's underground classic *The House of God*—"The delivery of medical care is to do as much nothing as possible"—epitomizes therapeutic nihilism, the belief that the medicine's role is to assist the body to heal itself, but the law applies equally well to testing. Students and residents are admonished to test sparingly, but what is to be spared? The patients' pain and inconvenience? Their money or time or fearful suspense? The staff's time and inconvenience? The hospital's or the HMO's money? The best critical path from differential diagnosis to diagnostic conclusion is not necessarily the shortest, and attempts to be expeditious risk premature closure. The goal is to avoid until necessary the invasive (and expensive) tests like CT scans and angiograms, technologies that have made obsolete not only "exploratory" surgery but also some of the older internist's subtle strategies of physical diagnosis and clinical reasoning. In the intellectual exercise that is internal medicine, a physician who lacks tact and judgment in testing strategy is not only wasteful and inconsiderate but inelegant, almost unsporting. Those who resort to CT scans when simpler tests or a good history and physical would serve as well risk their colleagues' scorn.

Nevertheless, when the diagnostic stakes are high or there is a strong likelihood that an invasive test will eventually be necessary, the usual prohibitions and cautionary advice are set aside. In these circumstances, the neglect of finer points of test-choice strategy in the single-minded pursuit of a diagnosis is likely to be justified by an appeal to Sutton's law. The eponym comes not from an honored clinical ancestor but from a criminal. Asked why he robbed banks, Willie Sutton is said to have replied: "That's where the money is."[27] The "law" is doubly interesting. It is unintended evidence of the carefully preserved fiscal innocence of academic physicians, who invoke Sutton's law even in a time of cost constraint without hearing the double meaning a critic of medical expenditure would find in it. More important as a part of a counterweighted pair of maxims is its appeal to an outlaw. Clinical reasoners could use instead the Sufi tale of Nasrudin or a "little moron" joke about searching for an object under a lamppost instead of where it was lost, but the choice of a bank robber implicitly acknowledges that the maxim to test sparingly has been violated. Like Sutton, physicians in this particular instance are outside the rules; like Sutton, they have their reasons. The maxim is elevated, unusually, compellingly, to a "law." That it is attributed to Sutton reminds physicians that, however goal-oriented and successful, their decision to opt for the quick diagnostic payoff ignores the clinical canons of technological restraint.

Diagnosis

Occam's razor, or
"Look for a single diagnosis that can explain all the findings"

"It's parsimonious, but it may not be right," or
Hickam's dictum

Reaching a diagnosis engages in the most practical way the tension between the welter of the phenomenal world and the patterns imposed on it by biological science and clinical experience. As the problem of the anomalous fact suggests, when a physician considers what the details of a patient's history and physical add up to, the number and complexity of signs and symptoms occasionally raise the possibility that two disease processes are at work instead of one. But, "Entities should not be multiplied unnecessarily," as William of

Ockham famously declared;[28] and Occam's razor, as this maxim is called, is the surgical instrument most favored by internists. Beginning diagnosticians are cautioned to resist the allure of comorbidity, a double diagnosis that can account for all the details of the patient's presentation. If a detail doesn't fit, the principle of parsimony will be invoked: there may be a different, better explanation for the whole. Physicians are admonished to look instead for a diagnosis that can account for all the signs and symptoms and all the test results.

But the quest for an elegant single solution is contradicted by the very real possibility, especially among the elderly and the poor, that one patient really does have two new diseases. As Hickam's dictum puts it (and in rhyme): "The patient can have as many diseases / As the patient damn well pleases."[29] Thus the physician's store of clinical wisdom must include, along with the details of improbable diagnoses that might fit the evidence, an awareness of a small but important chance of comorbidity. Like the rare disease, the possibility of two diseases emerging at once is to be considered only in cases of demonstrated logical need when all efforts to find a simpler, single solution have failed.[30] For a clinician, not to remember that misfortunes are sometimes multiple can be a source of embarrassment or, worse, diagnostic (and thus therapeutic) delay.

Treatment

"Relieve the symptoms."

"Make the diagnosis."

Treatment often resolves the tension that pervades the question of diagnosis, but it can pose problems of its own. The physician's task is to relieve suffering. But just as medicine's traditional maxim, "First do no harm," seems to be contradicted by the pain of testing and treatment, so the therapeutic imperative is sometimes constrained by the need to obtain a diagnosis. Good treatment depends on good diagnosis. The tension between the two duties can be seen in a case of serious infection. The symptoms are distressing— fever, chills, rigors, with the possibility of seizure—but if an antibiotic is given immediately there will be no chance to determine exactly which organism is causing the illness. The patient's recovery may be delayed and other people endangered. Broad-spectrum antibiotics provide some escape from this dilemma: what does the identity of the unknown agent of infection matter so long as it is eliminated? But here, as elsewhere in medicine, there is a trade-off. What is broad may be poorly focused: those antibiotics may not work as soon or as well as another that might have been chosen had adequate tests been done before the treatment began, and the consequences for others exposed to the disease also must be put into the equation. To philosophers, the word "empirical" designates the real-world, experience-based practicality characteristic of science. But in medicine, though it represents accurately the deduction from general law that is characteristic of science, "empirical" is the label for treatment prescribed without proof of diagnosis, the epitome of what medicine regards as "unscientific" practice.

A fairly common, more painful example of this tension between the alleviation of suffering and the diagnosis of the disease is created by the detection of widespread cancer from an unknown primary site. A biopsy is necessary to make the diagnosis, and therapy, "real" therapy targeted at the source of the spread, as distinguished from palliation of the symptoms from the secondary site, is impossible without a diagnosis. As residents sometimes say, "no meat, no treat." Will the therapy, itself also harmful, be effective enough to justify the pain of obtaining the tissue sample? Will it make a significant difference in the course of the disease? Careful analysis of the benefits and the burdens is called for, and a decision not to pursue the diagnosis almost always has an edgy, defiant feel to it. Geriatricians usually are far more comfortable than other physicians with forgoing diagnosis. They believe an elderly patient's functional status is more important than a test that may have only a marginal value.[31] Such tests include quite ordinary ones that may nevertheless disorient the patient, and their definition of "function" has even been broadened to include maintaining the patient's social support.[32]

Clinical education can highlight the potential conflict between diagnosis and the care of the patient. Clinical teachers face, farther along in the patient encounter, the tension between advice and example we saw with the review of systems. For example, the diagnosis of chronic arthritis separates patients into two categories: those with degenerative and those with inflammatory disease. The two forms of arthritis are distinct, and discriminating between them is essential for postresidency fellows studying to become rheumatologists. But tests may be expensive, time-consuming, or painful, and, at least in the initial states of therapy, the difference is immaterial for many cases and not immediately important for any. No matter which form of the disease the patient has, the treatment proceeds in slow stages from low doses of a relatively mild agent to higher doses, then to graduated doses of a stronger drug—and so on in ascending steps. The drugs prescribed for either form of the disease are initially the same. Not until fairly far along in the treatment of a recalcitrant case does it matter whether the arthritis is degenerative or inflammatory. Should residents and fellows be taught to diagnose the disease or to treat the patient? The answer, as with much else in medicine, is "both." This balancing act can be maintained over a practice full of patients or even through an afternoon's clinic. But when "both" is a logical impossibility, as it must be in the care of an individual patient, physicians habitually remind one another (and themselves) of the other, unchosen half of the contradictory pair. "You really need a diagnosis," they will say if the patient has been treated empirically. Or if the diagnosis has been pursued, "It's also important to treat the patient's discomfort." Whichever rule is followed, the other is likely to be invoked.

Situational Rules in Case-Based Reasoning

Aphorisms and maxims that guide the clinical encounter are the intermediate rules of medicine's clinical casuistry. Albert Jonsen and Stephen Toulmin, who note the similarity between case-based moral reasoning and clinical reasoning in medicine, define casuistry as

> the analysis of moral issues, using procedures of reasoning based on paradigms and analogies, leading to the formulation of expert opinions about the existence and stringency of particular moral obligations, framed in terms of rules or maxims that are general but not universal or invariable, since they hold good with certainty only in the typical conditions of the agent and circumstances of action.

In their definition, maxims are the "formulas drawn from traditional discussions and phrased aphoristically which served as fulcra and warrants for argument."[33] As part of the process of considering what in good conscience can be done in troubling situations, maxims serve to fit the prevailing wisdom—authoritative and experience-based but often unstudied—to the circumstances of a particular case under consideration.

Jonsen and Toulmin might have been describing the consideration of a medical case and the discursive clinical reasoning about what ought best to be done for a particular patient. In that clinical casuistry, physicians call upon their store of case-based practical knowledge: the paradigm or "classic" cases, along with cases known to them that, like the present one, depart from the paradigm in some recognizable way, and the aphoristic rules of thumb that summarize acceptable, customary practice in similar circumstances. Thus maxims and aphorisms are part of clinical judgment. They support the interpretive thinking that enables physicians to reason abductively from effect to cause and to fit a body of experiential, science-based knowledge to the predicament of a particular patient.

Because clinical knowing is uncertain, clinical teachers guide rational practice and encourage good judgment with clinical maxims. The tentative status of that reasoning is signaled by the informality of even the most dogmatic maxim and by the existence of its opposite, lying in wait for another, different case. Through their mutual contradiction, the opposed maxims remind learners faced with a difficult clinical question to consider the alternatives. The goal is not to find a middle way or a compromise between them but to choose the best—or least harmful—course of action in particular circumstances. Nevertheless, each of these maxims may be uttered as if it were the singular truth, and the physicians who invoke them by and large behave and teach as if there were no possible contradiction. By this means, teachers of clinical medicine may lay claim to science but hedge like racetrack touts.

Narrative and the Contextual Use of Contradictory Rules

There are good reasons for a rational science-using enterprise to use such contradictory maxims, but physicians apparently ignore them. A rationality that relies on contradictory rules seems unworthy of a profession that draws on science and aims at error-free efficacy. Skeptics could be forgiven for wondering how rational thinkers can use such folk wisdom seriously, especially to teach beginning physicians. When elders utter first one old saying, then soon after in another case its opposite, their pronouncements could easily be seen as mere simulacra of rules and dismissed as a quaint communal custom that will soon disappear. Yet these counterweighted situational rules embody the tension inherent in clinical knowing. They do not fit the prevailing view of medicine as a science; in fact, they undermine it. Uncertain circumstances and the lack of absolute rules do not ease the obligation to take action or the need for guidance.

The value of the contradictory maxims is rooted in the interpretive nature of clinical reasoning and physicians' focus on one patient at a time. Counterweighted, competing advice is neither accidental nor the remnant of a bygone era. The maxims work in the real-life care of patients and in clinical education precisely because of their contradiction. Diseases are not diagnosed and treated in test tubes but in human beings, where they develop variously over time; both diseases and patients are best understood in light of their histories. Those narrative accounts—the natural history of signs and symptoms that make up medicine's diagnostic plots, the history of this patient's present illness, the social history, the family history of disease—must be pieced together and interpreted to create the medical case that accounts for this episode of illness. Aphorisms and maxims, however wise and conclusive they may sound, were never meant for universal application; they are situational wisdom that has arisen out of (and proven useful in) circumstances very like those identified in a particular case. The key to their value lies in the circumstances of their use and, within a single case, their timing. Thus when one half of an aphoristic pair suggests itself, its opposite may not only seem irrelevant but does not even come to mind.

A maxim is always case-based. It is contextual and interpretive, and its context is the patient's history of illness and medical attention, as well as the medical narrative of diagnosis and treatment. Subsequent observers may interpret events differently, and then a clinician who invokes an aphorism will very likely hear a physician of equal or higher rank invoke its opposite. Clinical reasoning is the interpretation of unfolding events rather than a process so exclusively visual and so devoid of time as the recognition of a "disease picture" or pattern. Maxims guide and test this interpretive task even in an era of algorithms. Diseases are developing plots rather than static objects; they are narrative patterns that complicate themselves and unravel contingently through time. Physicians must make sense not only of signs and symptoms but also of their progression. As they do, they factor in their sense of the stage of the investigation and the reliability of the information received thus far.[34] The interpretation (and the applicability of a maxim) may be interrupted, sidetracked, or overturned by altered circumstances, whether a new event or the discovery of something previously unknown.

When a 40-year-old man comes to the emergency room slurring his words and "unlike himself," the cause is not immediately clear. But because his sister had a stroke at 40, stroke is strongly suspected in his case too. Nuclear magnetic resonance imaging (MRI) showed an enhancing lesion of the brain, and a neurologist was called. But the third-year student assigned to the case had a skilled cardiologist as his first clinical preceptor, and he thought he heard a heart murmur different from the innocuous systolic-ejection murmur the resident had recorded in the patient's chart.

"The neuro stuff on scans was way over my head back then," the student reported at the end of the year. "They were pretty sure his primary problem was neurological. But it made sense to me that he had a vegetation on one of his [heart] valves and it had gone to his brain." In the patient's chart he documented the murmur as he had heard it.

A number of clinical rules are at work in this case: one maxim promotes skepticism about the family history even as it is kept in mind as a major guidepost, and another calls for a review of systems despite the initial impression of stroke. Epistemological guidelines will help the student weigh the likelihood of stroke in a 40-year-old with a positive family history, the reliability of the MRI as a test specific for stroke, even the reliability of his own novice perceptions. The zebra aphorism "When you hear hoofbeats, don't think zebras," may be invoked: the hoofbeats are the brain lesion, but what is their most likely source? The student's documentation of the murmur was the detail that prompted (and supported) his working hypothesis that the patient's malady was not a stroke but an infection seeded from heart to brain. When, soon afterward, the patient developed a fever, Occam's razor called for a wholesale reinterpretation of the case. The student's observation was highlighted, the patient was sent for an echocardiogram, and the diagnosis of endocarditis was quickly made.

As a clinical case, this account would be less interesting, scarcely narratable in fact, if the events of the patient's illness had been matched from the start with the well-established diagnostic plot of endocarditis that became the diagnosis. Instead, even though the diagnosis was soon made, for a brief time the illness was a puzzle. The case begins with mental status changes, but the story that unfolds is deceptive; the family history is a false lead, and even the MRI is something of a red herring. The "real" plot will not be clear until it has unfolded a bit further: more time is needed, more clues, a rival interpretation. There is into the bargain an interpreter who is young, skilled, and lucky in his selective ignorance. Is the primary diagnosis a cerebral hemorrhage, as the signs strongly indicate? Or, as yet unsuspected by anyone but the third-year student, is it a vegetation that has spread to the brain from the slightly noisy heart valve? This is the case-based suspense of clinical medicine. In the interpretive, plot-detecting effort that constitutes diagnosis, competing maxims govern the process of fitting symptoms to the disease taxonomy and then determining how best to treat the patient. That all maxims have their opposite encourages in students and physicians a practical skepticism that prompts them to question their expectations, interrupt patterns, and see new forks in the road as the case unfolds. Only after the fact can the diagnostic options be seen as static patterns or algorithms.

If clinical reasoning were simply a matter of pattern recognition or follow-ing an algorithm, a well-programmed computer might substitute for even the best physician. But the accumulated and contradictory wisdom distilled in clinical maxims reflects the importance of time and context in the work of clinical perception and interpretation. That wisdom is honed by the case-based nature of medical practice and the narrative rationality good patient care requires. Like adages in general, good clinical maxims have their opposites. Their contradiction is central to the case-based reasoning that constitutes clinical judgment. By means of a collection of apparent paradoxes, students and residents are taught (and experienced clinicians reminded) to balance both sides of difficult judgment calls. In spite of the claim that medicine is a science, clinical education manages both to acknowledge the inescapable uncertainty of clinical knowing and to encourage habits of rational practice. The means are represented most succinctly by the contradictory maxims that guide and teach clinical judgment.

CHAPTER EIGHT

⸻

"Don't Think Zebras":
A Theory of Clinical Knowing

> Virtues necessary for practical rationality
> require initiation into communities and
> traditions and their attending narratives.
>
> —ALASDAIR MACINTYRE

CLINICAL MEDICINE SHARES both its epistemological predicament and its rational method with history, economics, anthropology, and the other human sciences—all disciplines less certain than the physical sciences and far more concerned with meaning. Unlike those disciplines, medicine does not reflect on (because it does not readily acknowledge) its interpretive character or the intermediate rules it uses to reach its conclusions. Instead, claiming a "technical rationality"[1] based on science, medicine takes little notice of either the tensions inherent in its practical reasoning or the ingenious means it has devised for expressing and mediating those tensions. Chief among these are the competing and counterweighted but thoroughly commonsensical maxims and aphorisms described in chapter 7.[2] In uncertain circumstances, they guide the real-life clinical rationality that is ignored or misdescribed in the profession's claim to be (or to be on its way to becoming) an old-fashioned positivist science.

Medicine also relies on counterweighted maxims—more general ones— for a comprehensive theory that can account for both its scientific knowledge and its practice. Despite its scientific basis, medicine has no overarching rule or theory of knowing that can resolve the tensions inherent in practice.[3]

Clinicians, however, do have some metarules, and together these generalizations serve as an ad hoc theory of clinical knowing. Like the more particular maxims that guide the clinical encounter, they turn out to be aphorisms and other traditional nuggets of wisdom. And, like them, each one can be uttered like dogma and still be contradicted by another metarule of equal weight and counterforce. They represent both the means by which physicians know what they know and their contradictory but practical way of teaching and refining clinical rationality. Taken together, these metarules are medicine's theory of knowing in practice: not an epistemology but a phronesiology of clinical medicine.

"Don't Think Zebras"

"When you hear hoofbeats, don't think zebras" may be medicine's chief interpretive rule. As medicine's epidemiological watchword, it reminds clinicians that the presence of signs and symptoms shared by a number of diagnoses is not likely to indicate the rare one on the list. Useful advice in itself, the zebra aphorism epitomizes the practical reasoning used by physicians in the never wholly certain task of caring for sick people. Like the maxims that guide the physician in taking the patient's history, performing a physical examination, ordering tests, and choosing therapy, the zebra maxim participates in a system of paired and competing rules. But it is unique in its solitary compactness. The epitome of medicine's counterweighted method of teaching and reinforcing the exercise of clinical judgment, "Don't think zebras" is a self-contained contradiction.

"But wait," a young clinician is likely to object, "Isn't that backward? Surely the advice is 'When you hear hoofbeats, *think* zebras.'" As a matter of fact it's not, but the reversal is instructive, almost as interesting as the aphorism itself. Far from suggesting that such old saws should be ignored as either the trivial pleasantries of a scientific discipline or the unavoidable byproducts of grueling work at the borders of life and death, its reversibility illustrates the use of counterweight and contradiction in negotiating the tensions of clinical practice. But unlike the paired maxims that guide the clinical encounter, the zebra maxim lacks an opposite. Instead, it generates its own competing rule.

The injunction *not* to think about zebras is strange enough. Even for a generation that learned about bad guys from crime drama instead of westerns, hoofbeats prompt the idea of horses. Zebras represent the rare to locally nonexistent occurrence. Why would a clinical instructor waste good breath advising, even commanding, a novice physician to think obvious, ordinary thoughts and not think unusual ones? In part, the answer lies in medicine's thoroughness in the face of uncertainty. As a practical intellectual activity on which life and health can depend, clinical medicine prides itself on taking into account every possibility. Consequently, when a set of symptoms is presented to medical attention, the ordinary is not necessarily the most obvious explanation. Reputations, even whole careers at the pinnacle of academic medicine, depend on thoroughgoing familiarity with and rapid recognition of the various maladies in a clinician's chosen field. Anyone can diagnose a sinus infection. Experts are known by their ability to diagnose Wegener's granulomatosis or to distinguish allergic bronchopulmonary aspergillosis from ordinary asthma. The question in academic medicine thus becomes why an aspiring young physician would *not* want to think about the zebras.

The answer is plain: rare diseases are rare. They are so rare that the likelihood of any given physician on any given day finding himself or herself in the presence of rare disease is exceedingly small. When the physician hears hoofbeats, even when he or she also glimpses some distinctly odd markings, it is far more likely that a horse has taken on another color or that the observer does not know quite everything there is to know about horses. Nevertheless, rare diseases do occur, and both the content and the character of medical education are skewed by the fact that academic medical centers are metaphorical savannas, zoological refuges for difficult-to-diagnose maladies of every stripe. Thus students and residents learning medicine see zebras far more frequently than do most practicing physicians. The clinical aphorism "Don't think zebras" is meant to remind clinical apprentices of the ordinary, real-world epizoology that not only awaits them outside the teaching hospital but also, despite the relative frequency of rarities there, still prevails within it. Even in a tertiary-care medical center, as another tongue-twister of a saying has it, "Uncommon presentations of common diseases are more common than [common presentations of] uncommon diseases."

Test questions, however, present medical students and residents a different, nonepidemiological set of probabilities. Because thoroughness is a clinical virtue, learners are expected to know far more than the easily recognized, common maladies. "What's the differential for shortness of breath?" a clinical teacher will ask. The peripatetic pop-quiz customarily carried on during a morning's work in an academic hospital includes questions by superiors that can range over the full list of diagnostic possibilities. The young are expected to be able to construct that set of possibilities—a differential diagnosis—for all sorts of signs and symptoms and then to whittle down the list by ruling out the least probable. In response to such pressure, students and residents customarily invert the zebra aphorism. To remember the unusual, the odd, and the rare is good advice for anyone who hopes to impress a senior resident or an attending physician with a long differential and prompt rule-outs.[4] The written tests at the end of student clerkships and, emphatically, the specialty board examinations that loom at the end of residency reinforce this inversion; and in hospitals where the nail-'em-to-the-wall custom of pseudo-Socratic questions called "pimping" prevails, "Think zebras!" is essential advice for daily survival.[5]

Useful as the statistically improbable may be to the young, however, the genuine clinical aphorism warns *against* thinking zebras, and it is worth examining for what it reveals about both clinical medicine and the practical education of physicians. The zebra aphorism is particularly valuable in understanding the cultivation of clinical judgment.[6] Day in and day out, whether in an academic subspecialty or in a primary-care practice, physicians must balance their knowledge of the whole realm of interesting medical possibility with a firm grasp of the statistical probability of any part of it. This task, well carried out, constitutes the exercise of good clinical judgment that is every physician's goal. To this end, the aphorism "Don't think zebras" enjoins learners and experienced clinicians alike to put to careful use what they know of statistical probability. It cautions them, when faced with a singular, ill-fitting bit of evidence, to assume that the cause is not a rare disease but one statistically more likely. "When you hear hoofbeats," therefore, "don't think zebras."

Still the zebras are there, unforgotten, unforgettable, right there in the aphorism. Not only does the advice generate its own counteraphorism among the young but also, as a reminder to forget, it is contradictory in itself. As long as the injunction not to think zebras comes to mind, zebras cannot be unthought. Physicians think zebras even as they remind themselves not to. The maxim captures in a nutshell medicine's skeptical recognition of competing, potentially contradictory interpretations of essential signs and the competing, potentially contradictory choices that are based on them.

This paradoxical maxim is the epitome of medicine's practical rationality, its quintessential interpretive rule. Because the management of uncertainty in all its variety is the central, if never quite stated, theme of clinical education, the self-contradiction of the zebra maxim teaches commonsense procedure in a field where improbabilities should not be forgotten, even as they are not actively considered. Acknowledge them, implies the aphorism, even as you set them aside. Their wild presence should be pursued only if they represent an immanent danger; otherwise, they should be ignored in favor of more obvious possibilities. In the care of the ill, such balance is important. A physician must not forget the rare and catastrophic possibilities, but, if the patient is not in immediate danger, the most likely diagnosis must be attended to first. Distant possibilities will come to attention only when the obvious and common are eliminated.

This practical wisdom is all the more important because most North American medical schools teach clinical medicine in tertiary-care hospitals. Special arrangements must be made to give students and residents the everyday experience of primary-care office practice. The difficult pedagogical task is to educate new physicians (and sustain good practice in experienced ones) despite the constant potential presence of rare conditions. Because medicine cannot discard or ignore its outliers, it needs a way to restore their proportionate importance. It must both reward the recognition and timely treatment of rare diseases and remind even subspecialists that rarities are not the stuff of medical practice, not even in an academic medical center. The zebra rule does just this. In situations of uncertainty—and every case, whether easily apprehended or strikingly unusual, is capable of surprise—the zebra aphorism embodies the wisdom of accumulated experience: no matter how unlikely, the improbable is possible but must not be allowed to skew the judgment. In full recognition of this, unless there is a possibility that endangers the patient, a physician attends first to the obvious and ordinary.

On Beyond Zebras: A Phronesiology of Medicine

The zebra maxim, like other clinical sayings, is widely used but almost entirely unexamined. This is not surprising, since it is part of the interpretive strategy—a theory of knowing in practice—that medicine relies upon but resolutely ignores. As a bottom-up rule of practical knowing, it is part of the phronesiology of medicine. "Phronesiology" draws on Aristotle's distinction between episteme and phronesis, two kinds of intellectual virtue, to designate a theory of practical knowing that is different from "epistemology," a theory of scientific knowing. Phronesiology, by contrast, is what we know about rationality in situated, contingent circumstances like moral quandaries or illness. Covering, universal laws can be generated for the sciences, but in other, more context–dependent fields such laws tend to be trivial or useless. Thus, the goal of phronesis or practical reason is not to determine a law-like answer that will apply to all such cases but to decide, on balance, the best thing to do in this particular circumstance.[7]

Like Edgar Allan Poe's purloined letter, medicine's phronesiology is a secret hidden right out in plain sight. The fundamental skill of the physician is to determine a treatable cause from the evidence of its effects, symptoms and signs that are sometimes unusual or transient. A thorough knowledge of human biology is essential, but it is not enough to accomplish the task. Medical students crammed to the gills with scientific information must learn to reason clinically, "backward," by identifying diseases from their bodily clues. This involves learning to perceive and to interpret what is perceived—sometimes (but not at every stage) separate matters. Students must also learn what questions to ask of patients, a skill that is less "natural" than it seems, and how to make sense of what they are told. This learning process is framed by scientific knowledge about how the body works at various levels: organ down to molecule. The goal is to fit all the information they gather—the patient's history and presenting symptoms, the perceived signs of illness, the test results—with all they know about the body and what can possibly go wrong with it. And this is just for the diagnosis. Treatment, although sometimes wonderfully simple and effective, can be complicated: allergies, side effects, drug interactions, effects on other conditions the patient may have, the patient's willingness and ability (too often in the United States a matter of money) to adhere to the most effective regimen. The task of prognosis is likewise vexed by therapeutic optimism, doubt about the relevance of statistics to the individual patient, a wariness of self-fulfilling prophecies, and the fear of death.[8]

Fortunately, clinical guidance exists: pathognomonic signs, recognizable syndromes, criteria for diagnoses, guidelines, protocols, algorithms. These are well established by tradition; some have also been confirmed by clinical research. Their solidity is a practical fact. Protocols are regularly given to nurses, physicians' assistants, and emergency medical technicians, and in clinical discourse dogma abounds. But beyond basic rules like "Airway, breathing, circulation" in the care of trauma patients, clinical guides do not have the universalizability or the force of physical law.[9] Medical practice lacks nonobvious rules that can be generally and unconditionally applied to every case, even every case of a single disease. The use of intermediate rules and algorithmic decision pathways take clinical students only part of the way.

When do such rules and guidelines apply and when should good clinicians ignore them? How should they interpret deviant or insufficient signs? When should they think outside the box? The long clinical apprenticeship is spent first learning rules and then learning their limitations and exceptions in particular circumstances. Luckily, by this time most clinical learners have forgotten the neat, conclusive expectations of medicine they had when they were science students and are laboring to meet the practical demands of their clinical instructors. This is not a simple forgetting: they are learning to perceive clinical matters like physicians. Their senses are as engaged as their minds. They learn physical signs with eyes and hands and ears and nose, even as they absorb the concepts of disease and therapy those signs entail. They want to be doctors: they want to be able to diagnose and treat patients. If the biology textbooks they devoured in the first two years now seem distant abstractions, it matters not a whit; evidence-based medicine gurus advise clinicians to burn their textbooks.[10] Instead, they are acquiring clinical maxims, rules of thumb, and tricks of the trade, along with instructions, habits, and skills from their clinical elders. Yet the working assumption all the while is that their clinical teachers' thinking is scientific: objective, testable, and potentially replicable in a series of similar patients. No matter how provisional the guidelines or how numerous the exceptions to them, they are imparted with the tacit assurance that once medicine is complete, the rules will be a set of certainties, a collection of self-interpreting algorithms.

As readers of signs, clinical students are also acquiring the judgment essential to an interpretive practice. The aim is a rigorous, intersubjectively replicable rationality, and counterweighted maxims play a part in teaching it. Far from learning an objective, contextless manipulation of facts, they absorb a set of interpretive guides and a sense of the situations in which to use them. Sometimes their thinking (and usually that of their teachers) is rapid, easy, even "automatic," as if they have achieved the formal sets of laws and procedural rules that might characterize an invariant and certain science.[11] Yet, as they work to identify causes for the effects they observe, they must take account of and accommodate the uncertainties of diagnosing and treating illness in particular human beings. Just as there are aphorisms and maxims that guide the clinical encounter, so too there are larger interpretive maxims that guide the clinical mindset. On close inspection, these rules of interpretive practice, the phronesiological maxims clinicians use to theorize the way they negotiate meaning and determine a course of action, are also paired and counterweighted, always competing, and often entirely contradictory.

The Goal of Clinical Medicine

> The therapeutic imperative, or:
> "Always do everything for every patient forever."
>
> *Primum non nocere,* or:
> "Don't just do something, stand there."

Every treatment decision takes place within a tug-of-war between the physician's pride of craft and a recognition of that craft's potential danger. For this reason and because the knowledge of those dangers is imperfect, medicine's therapeutic imperative is countered by the oldest of clinical maxims: *Primum non nocere;* above all, do no harm. Although both physicians and patients speak as if a drug's side effects could be separated from its therapeutic power, pharmacology is taught to medical students with almost as much emphasis on risks as on benefits. Likewise, a mutual suspicion is encouraged between residents in internal medicine and the surgical specialties as prima facie representatives of opposite poles of therapeutic response: dilly-dallying versus the quick fix.

We identify medicine with the therapeutic imperative. That's where the miracles are: wonder drugs, emergency rooms, timely surgery. Once surgeons refused to operate on Jehovah's Witnesses who refused blood transfusion, but in the 1970s they began to try. More successful in the aggregate than expected, these acts encouraged the techniques of bloodless surgery and the development of blood extenders, advances that proved valuable not just to subsequent patients who were Jehovah's Witnesses but to all surgical patients in the era of HIV infection.

But the therapeutic imperative is not invariably benign. Social forces sometimes tip the balance between activism and restraint and obscure the rational choice. Fear of malpractice litigation has kept obstetricians attached to the use of electronic fetal monitors in normal, uncomplicated childbirth—surely an occasion for minimalism—although studies have shown they do not achieve their intended effect of preventing cerebral palsy and lead to unnecessary Caesarian sections.[12] Likewise, the hope of cure (or fear of death) can prompt patients to choose extreme, go-for-broke treatment, even when a more moderate choice might do as well and leave them eligible for new treatment in the future. Consulted for a second opinion by a man about to undergo a treatment with a poor survival rate, Jerome Groopman interprets his test results as an insufficient confirmation of the diagnosis and, with difficulty, persuades him to accept symptomatic therapy instead. Groopman tells of going head to head with the diagnosing physician, who is certain that the patient will die of this neglect. To make matters more interesting, the patient is a scientist accustomed to solid proof, something that neither his original physician nor Groopman can give him. His choice is finally not between treatments but between physicians: he prefers Groopman's open assessment of uncertainty to the first doctor's assertion of authority. He recovers, and his puzzling symptoms are never explained.[13]

The tension between doing everything and doing nothing, particularly for people nearing the end of a terminal illness, has been scrutinized in medical ethics over the last three decades. In the 1970s, *The House of God* caught the conflict as technology first brought it to crisis: the hospital of the title, fount of healing miracles, is headed by men trained heroically to give their all. But clean water, good nutrition, and a century without war on this continent have combined with medical science and technology to yield a cohort of old people whose selfhood dies well before their bodies stop. At the heart of Shem's satire is the Chief of Medicine's once noble credo: always to do everything for every patient forever.[14] Since the 1970s, medicine and the society that holds it in such regard have learned that therapeutic limits are not the possible but, at times, the absurd. The therapeutic imperative rightly remains central to medicine. But against a narrow, purely technological understanding of the need to act, clinical teachers now occasionally intone a new maxim, itself a counterweighted inversion, that is the de facto motto of geriatricians and palliative care physicians: "Don't just *do* something," they advise. "Stand there."

The Use of Narrative in Clinical Reasoning

"Avoid the anecdotal."

"Pay attention to stories."

The counterweighted tension in clinical thinking is most visible in the conflicting wisdom about anecdotes as a source of clinically useful information. Despised and ignored by academic medicine, narrative accounts of individual instances are regarded as an aid to memory at best but red herrings of misleading personal experience at worst. Anecdotes are a diversion that may lead the unwary listener (and certainly the teller) astray. This disrepute now extends to the case reports that once made up much of the substance of clinical journals. Statistics made possible by larger collections of data are unquestionably more reliable than the single instance, and projects like the Cochrane Collaboration's database of systematic reviews and the American College of Physicians' ACP Journal Club reconcile diversely framed studies into more reliable aggregations of information that can guide medical decision-making, especially decisions about treatment.[15] Good clinicians are expected to use them and to work toward the elimination or minimization of narrative in diagnosis and treatment.

Anecdotes are nevertheless told—and, more than that, they are put to use in reasoning about problematic cases.[16] This is not likely to change, even when reference to the Cochrane analyses becomes an everyday part of clinical work. Indeed, the variation of the single case is the starting point for the EBM project. Valuable though epidemiological studies are, aggregated information constitutes generalized knowledge that must be applied to a particular patient. She may be younger than the groups studied—or more athletic or a vegetarian; she may be from a different ethnic group or have a late onset or a parent with the same condition. How and to what degree the studies apply in different circumstances is itself an occasion for comparative clinical storytelling, even among clinicians who know the prior probabilities for the Bayesian analysis of every malady in their specialty. The authors of *Evidence Based Medicine* know this. They advise clinicians to start with a question about one of their patients, research it as well as current studies allow, not only as a way of deciding what should be recommended to the patient but also to test and improve their clinical judgment.[17] From such particular cases will come the ideas for further epidemiologic and clinical investigation.

Good clinicians know what studies in case-based reasoning in cognitive science and medical informatics have corroborated: stories will never be eliminated from medical practice, not even from a thoroughly enlightened medical practice.[18] The status of the anecdote is much like that of the patient's history: taken for granted, the object of suspicion when brought to attention, but finally essential to the care of patients and ineradicable from practice. Although always potentially misleading, accounts of single instances in an uncertain domain continue to be cautionary reminders of exceptions to the rules. Thus, when anecdotes have sustained sufficient attack in a single conference or over time on a service, a seasoned clinician may remind colleagues and students, "Still, you can't ignore the stories."

The seductive oddity of a single instance should be enough to justify medicine's suspicion of narrative, yet the idea that medicine is (or can be) a science is used to back it up. The assumption is that physicians should use a top-down, scientific rationality that starts from biological "laws" and works deductively to apply them to the individual case. This is not how clinical medicine works, and if it were, it would truly be the "cookbook medicine" physicians dread. Worse, it would often endanger patients. But somehow this does not diminish the appeal of science as an ideal. Because the day-to-day diagnosis and treatment of sick people is an interpretive process, physicians go on relying on the narrative organization of details in a reasoning process that starts "bottom-up," or inductively from the particulars, and then circles between those particular observations and general rules, fitting the details to the patterned whole and testing the details in light of the known generalities. This is the rationality that C. S. Peirce called variously "abduction" and "retroduction" and described as essential to the retrospective reconstruction of cause from effect.[19] It is a practical, interpretive way of knowing in an uncertain world, a method shared by detectives, historians, hunters, readers, and (often) real-life, unidealized scientists. Anomalies—"clues" and the stories they generate—are vitally important to the process.

The Use of Experience in Clinical Knowing

"The research shows . . ."

"In my experience . . ."

These prefatory phrases often herald weighty clinical pronouncements by experienced elders, and while they may not look like rules for clinical reasoning, they draw on strong and potentially contradictory assumptions about the grounds of reliable knowledge. Each is likely to be invoked (perhaps on different occasions by the same physician) when discussion has gone too far in the direction of the other.

Clinical experience and research can be depicted as the two poles of medicine's practical knowing. But a closer view reveals clinical knowing as a continuum: vivid particulars burned into an individual memory at one end, the abstracted data summarized in the tables of published research at the other. Neither functions well without the other. Experience is the ground of medicine's rules of practice, and research flows from it. First there is a physician's own practice and its consequences, then that of colleagues, observed or reported, then journal reports of the experience of other clinicians, and the aggregations of clinical research. The Cochrane Collaboration and evidence-based medicine projects have added another layer of generalization, one that aims to render the variability of research studies commensurable and thus more usable, more reliable. Always, however, clinicians test the research results against their experience with their own patient population. A physician's judgment is shaped and goes on being refined by the continued interaction of experience and research.

Given that physicians receive a rigorous premedical introduction to science and a medical education that begins with two years of intense study in biology, we might expect that, even for those who do not pursue research careers, scientific studies will always outweigh experience. Surely physicians will adopt the new and well-tested therapeutic regimens and abandon ones that have been found inferior. All that is needed to alter diagnostic algorithms or introduce better therapies, one would assume, is wide publication of clinical studies. That, however, has proven not to be the case. Antibiotics, for example, do not affect most upper respiratory infections because those illnesses are usually viral; and because overuse eventually decreases the efficacy of antibiotics, their use for viral illness is useless for the patient and harmful for us all. But physicians go on prescribing them for colds and sore throats. Habits—rarely venial, sometimes sensible, but most often just reflexively conservative—prevail. This is especially true with regard to treatment options when published studies go beyond refining the current standard of practice to challenge it entirely. When hormone replacement therapy (HRT) was believed to lower the risk of osteoporosis and heart disease for postmenopausal women, few began HRT and few of them continued it for long.[20] Likewise, lumpectomy with radiation was long ago demonstrated to be as curative as mastectomy, but radical surgery went on being the treatment of choice for years. Physicians may be scientifically educated, but they also have responsibility for other people's lives. Their responsibility is exercised under conditions of uncertainty in a changing field of knowledge. No matter how sound a generalization may seem to be, exceptions inevitably arise. In such circumstances, therapeutic caution is so well founded that in characterizing new regimens in the second sentence of this paragraph, I used the word "well-tested" and not "proven." We know what "well-tested" means, but the criteria for "proven," a distinction tobacco companies and creationists have taken advantage of, are more difficult to meet.

Some of this caution is justified. Conclusions, like those about HRT, are often revised or subsequently limited in their implication. Patients differ: there are more and less suitable candidates for a treatment of choice. Skills also vary and the personal preferences of patient and physician may intervene. When given the choice between leaving a normal patient well enough alone or prescribing a medication with side effects that even for a very small number of patients will outweigh the acknowledged benefit, physicians are inclined toward errors of omission rather than commission. This may have been the situation with HRT, which was always known to increase the risk of uterine cancer slightly. Yet the therapeutic imperative, especially in life-threatening situations, can outweigh information from sound research, and confidence in their own experience may make physicians reluctant to alter, for example, habits of practice in an intensive care unit.[21] The strength of experience works against newfangled strategies like evidence-based medicine as well.

How do physicians acquire their habits of practice? The traditional Flexnerian division of medical education into scientific and clinical halves was originally designed to introduce clinicians to science, but now it marks the struggle to turn students of science into physicians capable of making wise decisions under conditions of uncertainty. This daunting pedagogical task traditionally is undertaken abruptly in the third year of medical school without any discussion of the character of medicine's rationality. After struggling to recast the biomedical sciences in terms of the care of sick people, every physician understands that scientific knowing is not the same as clinical knowing. They may choose to honor their profession by calling it a science, but they quite reasonably resist efforts to dislodge what their experience has suggested is efficacious. Equally reasonably, the profession as a whole counterbalances this conservatism with the injunction to "keep up with the research." Good clinicians know both what the studies show and what their own experience has been. Both are valuable. In good clinical practice and the theory of evidence-based medicine, each is shaped by the other.

The Nature of Clinical Knowing

"Medicine is a science."

"Medicine is an art."

The overarching paradox of medicine's theory of knowledge—or perhaps the fundamental one—is the one considered in chapter 2, the habitual description of medicine as both a science and an art. As a practice, medicine is neither, but the paradox stands for medicine's recognition of the importance of phronesis, the practical reasoning put to work in response to a sick person's request for help. Patients come to physicians for recognition of their predicament, identification of their malady, and action on their behalf. They want some idea of what lies in store as a consequence of both diagnosis and treatment. Although science has become essential to medicine in the last century, the unavoidable reality of its practice is the uncertainty of applying general rules to particular patients. As a result, while much of its knowledge is drawn from biological science, medicine at its best is exercised with an experiential skill that may feel or look like art.

The everyday practice of medicine takes place at the intersection of biological abstractions and the particular manifestations of disease in the individual patient. The tension inherent in negotiating uncertain possibilities is the inescapable consequence, and this is the starting point for clinical knowing. Although they are rarely addressed directly, this uncertainty and the ways of negotiating it are the constant preoccupation of clinical education. Clinical education seeks to equip and sustain physicians in the face of the inescapable uncertainty of their knowledge. They need both to know the scientific and clinical regularities and to stay open to the odd improbability. The image of medicine as a developing or "youngest" science is an attempt to account for this.[22] Good clinicians must recognize the authoritative order of things, including the importance of statistical data and the findings of evidence-based medicine. At the same time, they need to recognize the singular, unexpected event that is narratively organized and remembered and to evaluate its potential importance for practice. That is the achievement of the Dublin zookeeper, who successfully bred lions in captivity because he understood lions: every lion is different.

This crazy balance, a kind of double mindset, is not quite impossible to sustain. It is a stimulus for research in clinical medicine and, especially in difficult cases, the ballast of good patient care. Like good clinical judgment as a whole, the competing, often contradictory wisdom about the nature of knowing in medicine enacts the tension fundamental to clinical practice and to the education its practitioners receive.

Counterbalancing as a Practical Theory of Clinical Rationality

Beyond its traditional division into "basic science" and "clinical" halves, medical education takes little note of the mismatch between generalizable scientific knowledge and its particularizing practical rationality. The third and fourth years of medical school, followed by internship and residency, are often referred to as "training." The term is deplored as behaviorist and anti-intellectual by some clinical teachers, but it marks the difference between lectures, laboratories, and examinations in human biology and the learners' long, slow stages of apprenticeship to those above themselves on the educational ladder. Along with acquiring readily testable information, apprentices learn how to judge, how to act, how to conduct themselves as physicians. It is a matter of balancing competing claims. Beyond the classroom, after the last science exam is passed, in hospitals and clinics where they are increasingly responsible for the care of sick people, there are fewer invariably right and generalizable answers (although there are certainly wrong ones). Instead of answers, clinical education provides a preparation for practical, ethical action: how to respond, what best to do, how to discover enough to warrant taking action, which choice to make on behalf of the patient.

Medicine resolutely ignores the contradiction between its claims to be a positivist science and its interpretive practice even as the potentially contradictory, but always situational, rules of practice enable physicians simultaneously to express and to negotiate the contradiction. Clinical discourse and educational methods are guided by these counterweighted rules and shaped by their tension. Believing two things before breakfast, as the use of contradictory maxims seems to require, is in practical matters a brilliant, invaluable resource. Given that medicine's proverbial wisdom, like clinical practice itself, is always situational, always interpretive, it makes sense that its theory of practical reason is expressed in maxims that, even as they offer support for a way of knowing, can be countered by maxims that are their opposite. As lawyers, literary critics, historians, and other students of evidence know, rules are not self-interpreting. The maxims that theorize clinical knowing are relentlessly contextual and incapable of generalization to all similar cases, and with the exception of the zebra aphorisms, they come, like the maxims for the clinical encounter, in counterweighted and contradictory pairs.

Within medicine these counterweighted assumptions about the nature of knowing serve as clinical medicine's substitute for a comprehensive, reflexive account of practical reasoning and its uncertainties. Informal though they are, they constitute a theory of clinical practice, a phronesiology of medicine. They raise the question whether medicine, especially medical education, is well served by ignoring, as it does now, the counterbalanced tension of its rationality. Physicians have not objected to or investigated their odd pedagogical practice of guiding the young with potentially contradictory bits of advice. Is epistemological naïveté so useful that it ought not be disturbed? This visual field defect illuminates, as blind spots will, the assumptions of clinical knowing. It prompts us to wonder whether such obliviousness is valuable in itself and, beyond that, how self-conscious a physician's knowledge needs to be. Pretending that medicine is a science while working quite differently has served physicians well. If it ain't broke, maybe there's no need to know how it works.

Scholars in several disciplines testify that this obliviousness is common among practical reasoners. Hans-Georg Gadamer has observed: "Practice requires knowledge, which means that it is obliged to treat the knowledge available at the time as complete and certain."[23] Donald Schön in *The Education of the Reflective Practitioner* describes not only the automaticity of routine "knowing-in-action" but the execution of "smooth sequences of activity, recognition, decision, and adjustment without . . . 'having to think about it'" that is characteristic of "reflection-in-action."[24] Pierre Bourdieu, analyzing the interdigitation of culture and individual psychology in his concept of *habitus*, notes that a practice seems necessarily to "exclude from the experience any inquiry as to its own conditions of possibility." This "non-conscious, unwilled avoidance" leads him to find "the truth of practice [in] a blindness to its own truth."[25] Much the same "forgetfulness" undoubtedly lies behind the automaticity that Stuart Dreyfus, Hubert Dreyfus, and Patricia Benner have described as characteristic of expert knowledge.[26]

Those who have a visual field defect have no awareness of their lack. If practical knowing cannot know itself and practitioners are doomed to regard their knowledge as fixed and inviolable, then it may be futile to ask physicians or medical students to acknowledge either their rational method or their ingrained reluctance to acknowledge it. Even this inquiry into medicine's visual field defect, the one you are reading, might be misguided. If physicians are like the centipede that could not think about how it walks without falling over, then the prevailing imprecise account of medicine as a science and its traditional, unexamined method of clinical education ought to be left well enough alone. Or, if immobility is not a threat, what if the idealism of medicine's science claim is necessary to keep physicians on their toes?

Still, it is hard to believe that experienced physicians, many of whom in conversation readily acknowledge the uncertainty of clinical knowledge and action, cannot cope with an understanding of their knowledge and its procedures. There is much to admire in clinical reasoning. The zebra maxim and the counterweighted rules of knowing are rational and ingenious ways of accommodating the uncertainty and circumstantiality of practice. Calling attention to the way physicians think and work could be more humane and more effective—to say nothing of more interesting—than the often heard commands to "be thorough" and "keep up with research." As a society we expect physicians to have as their primary goals the accurate diagnosis and effective treatment of their patients, and medical education exists to foster the development of sound clinical reasoning. Why shouldn't they also be curious about it? Physicians are duty bound to marshal all the certainty available to them. Over the course of a career, biomedical and clinical research will regularly move the boundary between what is certain and what is unknown. Old questions are reopened by increasing knowledge and, as we have learned in the last quarter century, by new maladies. Each physician's personal boundary between certain knowledge and what is unknown undergoes similar (and equally unexpected) shifts as a result of ongoing education and participation in a community of practice. An understanding of the rationality of clinical medicine would deemphasize memorization and refocus education on learning to learn and on preparing physicians to cope with such changes over a lifetime.

Far from leading students and residents to throw up their hands—"Who knows?"—at the first whiff of difficulty, I believe that there would be real benefits if clinical education included some attention to medicine's epistemological predicament, its phronesiology, and the use of competing maxims as interpretive strategies for coping with uncertain knowledge. Clinical uncertainty is rooted in the activity of knowing itself, and acknowledging this might reduce the appeal of subspecialty medicine as a haven from uncertainty's discomforts. Refocusing medicine's distorted definition of science might increase the number of clinicians interested in the analysis and improvement of every aspect of medical knowledge and practice—whether in laboratory science, clinical research, or epidemiological investigation.

In the meantime, however, patients are in no danger. Despite its visual field defect, the inability to see all it refuses to know about its knowing, medicine works quite well. The odd, counterweighted, situational maxims that theorize clinical knowing go on performing their explanatory and justificatory tasks. They introduce the young and guide the experienced in medicine's uncertain, conflicted universe of practice and enable them to negotiate its contingencies and contradictions. They are unlikely to be displaced by identifying them as the de facto theory of medicine's practical rationality.

Take-Home Lessons

Although clinical knowing is inescapably uncertain, clinical education is occupied with locating the least slippery grounds for clinical action. In teaching hospitals, daily attempts are made to condense practical lessons into memorable, transmissible nuggets. It's a little like an algebra class shucking off those pesky word problems so as to learn the useful rules of solving for x and y. Every pedagogical occasion in clinical medicine, no matter how speculative or inconclusive, strives toward a useful take-home message, and a chapter on the counterweighted tension inherent in a theory of clinical knowing ought not to be an exception. This is particularly true because that tension represents the judicious balance clinicians seek through the exercise of clinical judgment.

Here are two take-home lessons, and—no surprise—they are counterbalanced pairs. The first justifies the continual review of cases in clinical medicine's practical, Deweyan education:

> "Experience is the best teacher."

> "Learn from others' mistakes."

The second take-home lesson concerns a difficulty that comes with learning in a hierarchical discipline:

> "Pattern your practice on that of your clinical elders."

> "Question everything you are told and much of what you see."

Contradictory approaches to clinical learning not only are expressed in competing maxims but, above all, are enacted in habitual clinical practice. Thus medicine may proclaim science as its ideal, but its theory of practical rationality is rationally guided by its dependence on contradictory and situational rules. Just as the foundation of the universe in the Hindu fable Clifford Geertz retells is reported to be "turtles the whole way down," so in medicine's phronesiology, clinical judgment seems to be governed by aphorisms the whole way up.[27]

CHAPTER NINE

⌒

Knowing One's Place:
The Evaluation of Clinical Judgment

> The countless acts of recognition which are the small
> change of the compliance inseparable from belonging
> to the field . . . are both the precondition and
> the product of the functioning of the field.
>
> —PIERRE BOURDIEU

IF A KIND of visual field defect obscures not only medicine's knowledge of the nature of its knowing but also an awareness of that lack, how is clinical judgment evaluated? If medicine were only a science, physicians could establish their clinical competence by answering test questions correctly. But because it is a practice, its evaluation is a much more complicated exercise. I stumbled on this realization by chance when I invited second-year medical students in my "Sherlock Holmes and Clinical Judgment" seminar to attend a hospital case conference in internal medicine so they could observe residents and attending physicians solving clinical problems out loud.[1] Two years before, soon after the arrival of a new chief, the department had been organized into three "firms."[2] For its British originators, the word "firm" is a nonsports synonym for "team."[3] And while Americans hear its corporate, money-making connotations, the advantages of the new arrangement soon made "firm" seem, locally at least, an entirely different word.

The firm system divided the internal medicine faculty so that each of the three comprised a full complement of subspecialists, and, although each group soon took on its own character, in composition each was representative of the whole department. Students and residents were assigned to a firm with the expectation that its smaller size would stabilize relationships and improve teaching and evaluation. Even patients had a de facto assignment to a firm. If they returned to the hospital within the year, they had a good chance of being known to the intern and resident taking care of them and, within three years, some chance that someone among the house staff would be familiar with their previous hospital stay. The linchpin of this increased coherence of teaching, consultation, and patient care was a weekly hour-and-a-half-long conference during which residents, students, a regular cadre of attending physicians who led the firm, and relevant specialists recounted the diagnostic process and the treatment decisions for two of the week's most interesting cases. "Firm conference" rapidly became what grand rounds in simpler days used to be: the liveliest, most communal occasion of the academic week.

"There are rules," I said to the students who planned to attend. "Wear your white coats."

They nodded. Well into their physical diagnosis course by then, they regularly wore their short white jackets at least once a week.

"Leather shoes," I said, forgetting about leather sports shoes. They nodded nevertheless.

"And," I hesitated, "pay attention to where you sit."

"What kind of rule is that?" a particularly literal-minded student teased.

"It depends on the firm," I answered.

I couldn't then be much more specific. In general, I could tell them, they should sit near the back of the room where third-year students sat (also wearing short white coats but distinguished by the stethoscopes in their pockets). They'd see.

At the appointed time, four students appeared, resplendent: men in dress shirts and ties, women in skirts and stockings, all in white coats and serious shoes. The conference I chose for us to attend—I'll call it the North Firm—met in a room with a wide entrance at the back. But, as the students headed for the nearest back-row seats, I found myself signaling them to the opposite side of the room, one-third of the way forward. The general rule, "neophytes at the back of the room," I realized, would have to be revised, at least for this firm.

Because clinical medicine is not a science, knowing the biological and clinical facts that appear on tests is only a start toward being a good clinician. A world away from experimental laboratories, which have their own ethos and behavioral norms, physicians learn how to comport themselves in ways that exhibit an awareness of their knowledge and experience and signal their status as clinicians.[4] The firm conference seemed a good place to study this. The next week, as students described the projects they were undertaking for the seminar, I took on one of my own. I would generate some reliable rules—"Where to Sit at a Firm Conference"—and report the last day of class. Although slightly tongue-in-cheek at the beginning, my aim was to describe the hierarchical seating pattern we had encountered so that exceptions and variations could be understood and formulated on the spot.[5] This chapter, somewhat belatedly, completes my assignment.

Evaluating Clinical Judgment

Clinical education is finely calibrated to instill and reward the development of clinical judgment in the face of uncertainty. It is a moral education because it shapes habits of action in the real world. But there is no good single test of its quality. Clinical skills can be tested, and so can the retention of information, and both are essential. But evaluating how they merge in genuine clinical competence is more difficult. Gross measures of patient outcomes are equally misleading because the correlation between the exercise of clinical judgment and the patient's subsequent health is poor: poorly treated but healthy patients often make a good recovery; well-treated but seriously ill patients often die. Test-makers struggle to obtain some indication of how clinicians would act, including the grounds for their decisions, in uncertain situations. But the conditional "would" is the operative word with written tests. A number of specialty exams include an oral component so that examiners can observe the candidate's response under duress. But long before that, clinical students and residents are evaluated just as they will be through the whole of their careers: on subjective but communal perceptions of their care of patients and their competence at clinical reasoning. In his study of surgical residency, Charles Bosk describes the constant evaluative process that goes on in clinical education.[6] It is no different in internal medicine, the specialty that dominates every student's introduction to the care of patients and contributes to the training of a large proportion of nonsurgical physicians: both its own residents and, for an internship year, residents in specialties like neurology, radiology, psychiatry, and anesthesiology. Thus, the rituals and practices of internal medicine, although they may be modified in other specialties, are central to the clinical education of every physician. The hierarchy of knowledge and experience is tested and reinforced in everyday rituals like hospital conferences. There the acquisition of clinical competence is subjected to self-evaluation and measured by signs of the participants' willingness to accept responsibility for its quality.

Reading the Signs

Because the firm system apportioned students and residents in equal numbers and assigned faculty evenly by rank and specialty, each conference offered an opportunity to observe the seating choices made by a representative sample of those engaged in the activities of an academic internal medical service.[7] The identification of participants by academic rank was simplified by their clinical coats. In the years I made weekly observations, status was strongly marked at the hospitals not only by their length but by their color: students wore short white jackets (W), house staff long blue coats (B), attending physicians long gray ones (G). So well established was the custom that, until federal regulations decreed that coats be laundered by the hospital rather than at home, a sharp eye could distinguish interns from residents by their darker shade of blue.[8] The few exceptions to the hospitals' color-coding belonged to senior faculty who had arrived sufficiently advanced in their careers to buck the system. They continued to wear the long white coats that identify attending physicians in most other academic medical centers. Since this minor color confusion was readily corrected upon glimpsing gray hair or an older-than-35 face, the status of conference participants was quickly discerned, and their seating choice could be easily recorded.

Since the three firms met simultaneously, one conference was observed each week and its seating pattern charted. Although my informal observation had begun from the inception of the conferences, charting began well into the firm system's second year and continued for 18 months. The charting period included two academic transitional periods of June and July. Observation was spread evenly among the three conferences in the early months, but as the study progressed, I focused on the firms I'll call North and East, the two most variable conferences. Colleagues, including those aware of my interest, rarely took notice of my charting activity. The prevailing view of seating choice, voiced by one of the only two physicians who asked me about my project, seemed to be that no one really cares where a person sits: "You just sit where you're more comfortable." Such "comfort," of course, is a very subjective criterion. When I told a physician from another institution who had been recently promoted to associate professor my working hypothesis—that rank and level of expertise are visibly displayed through the seating choice of participants—she responded dismissively, "Oh, I just take a seat!" But then, self-consciously, she laughed.

Results: The Display of Hierarchy

Week after week, charts of seating choice exhibited a stable if never entirely simple pattern that exemplifies the following well-recognized general rule.[9]

1. *Professors up front, students at the back.* Although seating is not assigned and is never discussed, it is ordered by academic rank on a

front-to-back-of-the-room axis. Senior attendings sit at the front; residents come next; students are at the back of the room.

This pattern could best be seen in the relatively stable West Firm (fig. 9-1) although the scarcity of seats in its small, tiered auditorium and the difficulty of reaching the far right seats once the conference began regularly resulted in a blending of ranks in border rows:

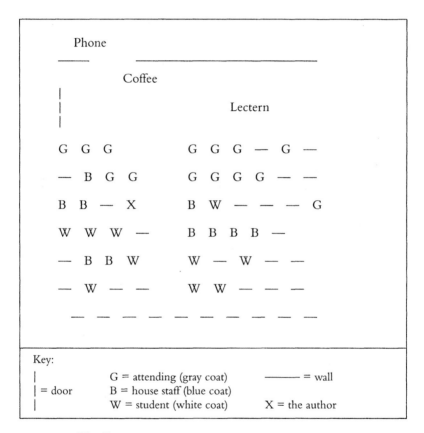

FIGURE 9-1. West Firm

The North and East firms, by contrast, met in larger, level, more accessible rooms that contained more chairs than usually were needed. These conferences regularly exhibited a lateral line of demarcation across the middle of the occupied seats. This de facto line separated the faculty from the young most clearly and consistently in the North Firm (fig. 9-2).

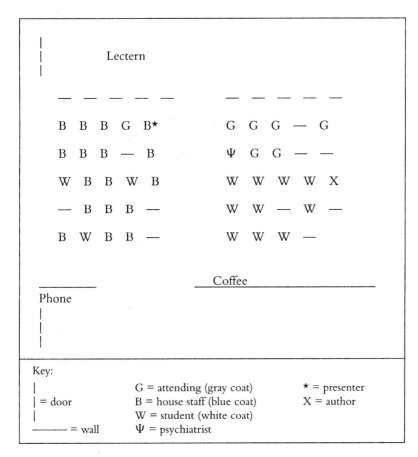

FIGURE 9-2. North Firm

The East Firm (fig. 9-3), often the best attended, showed the most variability, both in its settled patterns and in its weekly variation, but still exhibited a clear separation between faculty up front and students and residents at the back.

Exceptions Prove the Rule

The areas of unconformity in the North (fig. 9-2) and East (fig. 9-3) firms tested the tripartite, hierarchical, front-to-back distribution of participants: faculty first, then residents, and then students.[10] Although that general pattern was followed in both conferences, attendings avoided the front row, residents often sat at the back of the room, and students sometimes clustered toward the middle of one side or the other. Were these random variations that refuted

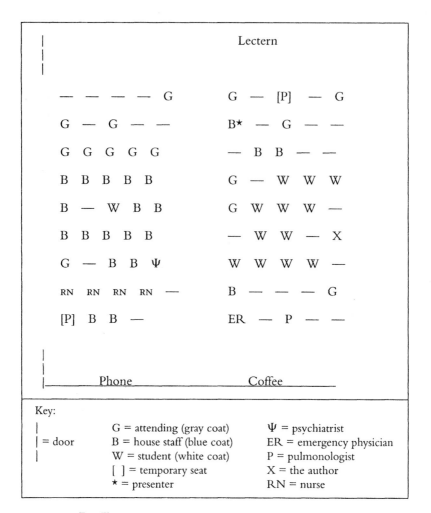

FIGURE 9-3. East Firm

the rule or did they follow some rule of their own? Further observation, far from disconfirming rule 1, refined it and made the strength of its operation clearer.

Attending physicians, who by reason of their rank, skill, and age are the most powerful people there, sat at the front of the room, but precisely where they sat was influenced by their relative rank and their anticipated importance to the cases to be presented. For residents (as I will show), there was the added influence of environmental features important for their work. In the West Firm, where seating was limited (fig. 9-1), attendings occupied the first row.

In the North and the East firms, which met in rooms with extra chairs (figs. 9-2 and 9-3), attendings left the first row empty. It seemed to be tacitly reserved for the chief of medicine and remained empty in his absence.[11] Whether beginning with the first row or second, patterns of seating choice in all three conferences produced a visible display of the academic hierarchy, physicians "in serried ranks assembled."[12]

Yet the rule was not followed with perfect strictness: an individual's seating choice might vary from week to week, and the borders between the groups—attendings, residents, students—could shift. Nevertheless, these variations were governed by observable factors. Younger faculty members made their choice—which is to say their distance from the front—according to their anticipated relevance to the cases on a given week. Residents, who enjoy the right of next choice, exercised it according to the construction of the conference room: the location and width of the entrance, the placement and relative privacy of the telephone, and the number and configuration of the chairs. Students, although they might mistakenly sit near a telephone the first time they attend a conference (but almost never, even the first day, at the front of the room), invariably worked out the pattern by the second week of their clerkship. They sat more or less together wherever the residents did not sit—unless they sat with the intern or resident to whose team they had been assigned.

In the two conference rooms that offered plenty of seating choice, then, the apparent exceptions to the strict rule of hierarchical seating added variety to the seating patterns. But because these variations were socially well controlled—known to all participants and regularly observed by them—the differences did not constitute violations of the general hierarchical rule. Indeed, they enforced the hierarchically ranked seating pattern while disguising its persistence. Thus, a senior attending, the acknowledged expert in his subspecialty, was able to claim with apparent sincerity that he sat up front "just so I can hear."

Some exceptions to the strict rule of seating by rank, themselves rule-like in their predictability, are as follows.

1A. *Sitting out of rank reinforces the hierarchical rule.* A person of any status may sit out of order in a higher rank—one rank only—if he or she is invited by word or gesture to do so or is presenting the case.

This rule applied especially to young faculty members whose subspecialty expertise had been summoned for that week's case. However new to the faculty, they regularly assumed a seat in a forward row—usually the second occupied row—with the expectation that they would justify their position before the conference was over. The exception also applied to students who occasionally sat with the interns and residents with whom they were working. Some latitude—quite literally—was also allowed to residents and students who were presenting one of the week's cases: they could sit farther forward than they otherwise would have. But the seat they chose, except in the restricted West conference room, was typically some distance from the center aisle. This lateral displacement, as I will show, signaled deference to the general rule.

Further inroads into other people's space have their rule, as follows.

> 1B. *Invitations may alter seating choice.* A person may sit more than one rank out of order if the host—whether resident, attending, firm chief, or the chief of medicine—sits with that person the entire time.

Caveat: This seldom happens. As soon as the host left, as he or she was almost certain to do, at least briefly to answer a page, the younger person was marooned in a forward row, visible to everyone in the room in his or her identifying coat—radiant white or glowingly blue. This seating option is best exercised by those out of the educational hierarchy: nurses who have taken care of the patient under discussion, the hospital lawyer, visitors from other institutions, or nonmedical guests who need never return.

> 2. *Peculiarities of the conference room may vary the pattern.* The configuration of the room—doors, telephones, location of entrance, number and mobility of chairs, and number of aisles shapes the pattern that becomes standard for each conference.

For me, the conference rooms came to seem like an electromagnetic force field, with the participants behaving like iron filings of various weights and densities. The peculiarities of each room were environmental phenomena that altered and sometimes redirected the flow of force in the following ways.

> 2A. *Access to the telephone influences residents' seating choice.* The placement of the telephone at the back of the room, as in the East and North firms (figs. 9-3 and 9-2), creates an area of unconformity. Where this occurs, the area nearby will be occupied predominantly, but not exclusively, by residents.

The tasks of patient care always trump educational ritual, including, when necessary, the observance of rank. In the North Firm, the conference visited by my second-year students, residents clustered at the back left, near the door (fig. 9-2). As a result, the dividing line was more sharply and more regularly drawn between the faculty thinly spread in the forward rows and students and residents in the last few rows, where they filled most of the chairs and typically did not save seats for those paged to the telephone. It was this well-established aberration that had motivated my sudden realization that the "right place" for my second-year students was halfway forward on the far side of the room, well out of the traffic of residents and latecomers. In the East Firm, too, where the telephone was located on the rear wall (fig. 9-3), a similar colonization took place; the back of the room, by rule a student area, frequently became the residents' space.

The West Firm had two telephones, one near the door and one in the hall just outside. The first, in an alcove more or less on stage, where every word was audible, was rarely used and then only by the very most senior attending physicians. The second phone in the hall was the instrument of choice and required residents to leave and reenter the room by the onstage door. Then they faced the problem of taking seats in the first row or moving very visibly father back: one sort of nonostentation struggled with another.

> 2B. *Latecomers and those who use hall phones sit near doorways.* The number, size, and location of entrances to a conference room govern the flow of those entering late or using the telephone. Latecomers and those returning from the telephone dive into the nearest available seats permitted by their status.

Not only did a single center aisle restrict the West Firm's small auditorium but also its relatively few seats were bolted to the floor in rising tiers. Its one door, "onstage" and parallel with the discussion leader and the case presenter (fig. 9-1), constricted movement further. Late entrances had to be made from stage right, and case discussions were regularly punctuated by frequent exits to the hall telephone. The privilege of sitting in the first row belonged to senior faculty, who, if paged, might claim any seat in that row on returning. Residents answering a page had to make the trek from middle seats, down the center aisle, out the onstage door, and back again by the same route. They did not have the option, as residents in other conferences did, of colonizing a few seats in a lower status area near the phone. If, on returning from the telephone, a resident occasionally decided to sit in the first row, he or she sat well forward in the seat, signaling a readiness to yield the position to a late-arriving elder.

In the East Firm, which met in a room with a forward door that was used (at least occasionally) by attendings, the customary front-to-back gradation was much less sharp (fig. 9-3). Or, to put it another way, the placement of doors gave the lateral position of a participant's choice more force. Students at the East Firm conference tended to sit across the room near the windows, faculty on the side near the doors. Residents occupied both halves but sometimes sat farther forward on the window side in the absence of a full clustering of faculty there.

>   2C. *Refreshments do not alter the pattern.* Coffee, fruit, muffins, and bagels, although highly valued by conference participants of every rank, do not affect seating choice. Over the 18-month period, several kinds of muffins and bagels were randomly introduced without discernible effect.

After scooping up food and drink upon entrance, participants in the North and East firms turned away from the table spread at the back of the room. Latecomers could avail themselves of refreshment, and persons of some standing might occasionally return for seconds, but no one in any conference ever was observed choosing to sit near the food. Indeed, in the West Firm, where refreshments were "onstage" next to an overhead projector, there were sometimes leftovers.

Variation within Ranks

Additional variations, especially within the three groups—faculty, residents, and students—are governed by clear rules that nevertheless work out differently each week, as follows.

>   3. *Lateral position is a secondary power gradient.* Seats on the center aisle outrank seats near the wall.

The power distribution between center and margins had nothing like the force of the front-to-back gradient. Its weaker force was evident in the fact that the middle seats between center aisle and wall were all but unranked. A seat on the aisle asserted more rank than one farther in, and a seat next to a wall suggested a bit of humility, especially if it was chosen before the room filled. But even in the North and East firms, chairs were not unlimited, and from week to week chance asserted itself.

As with the other hierarchical seating rules, the center-to-margin gradient was subject to variation within the prevailing pattern of a particular conference room. For example, in the West Firm, where a scarcity of seats forced choice, one might expect that less significance would accrue to choosing an aisle seat. But because the only passage was the center aisle, junior participants were unwilling to impose the inconvenience of squeezing down the row on their superiors, and thus the lateral ranking was actually somewhat stronger than in the other two conferences. In the North and East firms, the middle seats in each of the room's two lateral halves were the place for a sleep-deprived or poorly prepared resident to hide, surrounded by peers who by their eye contact might become more likely targets for the firm chief's questions. In the West Firm, by contrast, residents who hoped to disappear headed for the last row where, sitting with students, their feet were roughly at the presenter's eye level.

Although in the level rooms of the North and the East Firms there was a tendency for the half of the room closer to the door to outrank the half farther from it, this was probably explained by the position of the telephones near the door. Despite temporary preferences for aisle seats on one side or the other, over time in the North and East firms, neither side of a center aisle obviously outranked the other.

4. *Gender is overridden by status in the hierarchy.* Gender has relatively little effect on seating choice—even to a skeptical observer aware of the history of discrimination in medicine and in society at large.

The firm conference was a playing field of comfortable size upon which women residents and faculty could and did display their diagnostic and patient management skills. Women faculty knew the rules for seating and speaking, and they asserted themselves according to the expectations of their rank. Women residents did likewise. Women students often sat together in something of a "student section," but the fact that they were women did not seem to influence where they sat within the student group. My impression that men students sat more frequently with their residents and that women residents more often included students of both sexes in their seating group—and the potential effect of this difference, if substantiated, on residency choice and women's recruitment into academic medicine—might reward investigation.

5. *Individual exceptions prove the rules.* Regular attendees outside the departmental hierarchy (or with anomalous places within it) might be expected to disregard prevailing customs but instead establish habitual seating choices that express their position within the symbolic grammar of the prevailing seating pattern.[13]

Each conference included one or more regular attendees who were "outsiders." They might be clinicians from other departments regularly invited to attend and contribute their expertise, or they might be nonclinical members of the department of medicine. Where they sat was instructive, because it served as an ad hoc test of the seating rules that confirmed the meaning and importance of place. While at first glance the seating choices of these "outsiders" might seem to cut across the prevailing pattern, on closer observation, their location took the unwritten rules into account. Each person's anomalous situation was expressed in his or her location with the hierarchical order and its local variants.

The North Firm, for example, included a psychiatrist who attended regularly, asked questions that highlighted the psychosocial aspects of a case, and several times a year presented videotaped interviews with a patient under discussion. His regular seat was on the aisle halfway forward on the side of the room farthest from the door (see fig. 9-2). More often than not, his was the last row of the well-demarcated faculty section. That half of the room was, if anything, the less powerful of the two, but he took its most prominent seat. By contrast, the psychiatrist who only occasionally attended the East Firm sat toward the front when he knew he would be asked to contribute; otherwise, he sat near the back, scanning his mail, in the area of nonconformity chosen by latecomers and residents using the telephone.[14] In either place, he was on or near the aisle (see fig. 9-3).

The associate director of the emergency medicine division, who attended the East Firm conference, chose an anomalous seat that expressed his specialty's restless containment as a division in the Department of Medicine. He sat invariably in the aisle seat of the last row, pushed his chair back, and folded his arms across his chest as he listened (see fig. 9-3). That this place was left empty in his absence was perhaps at first due to the abundance of chairs in the room, but over time could be attributed to his frequent occupancy. The entire row eventually became "his": faculty members and residents who sat there seemed to be allied with him. Its out-of-order location expressed the energy he devoted to the customary tug-of-war on questions of diagnostic procedure between the emergency room and "the floors."

Almost as unorthodox were the seating habits of a young attending in pulmonary and critical care medicine (see fig. 9-3). Partly because her frequent contributions to the conference involved examining x-rays at the front of the room, but also because she had a somewhat ambiguous status as an assistant professor who was nevertheless an acknowledged expert, she often sat in three or four places during a single conference—none of which (until she read an early draft of this chapter) was in the well-occupied second row. It was as if she had been signaling a continuing recognition, despite her frequent prominence, of her somewhat lower status, but by the third year of the conference she had assumed the second-row position that she had steadily been earning.

And I? Even nonclinicians have their place at a hospital conference and need to know it. In all three conferences, I regularly sat near the far wall in the last faculty row. In the North Firm, this was one row in front of those seats toward which I had hastily redirected the second-year students (see figs. 9-1–9-3). "Professor," I imagined this seat declared, "though, of course, clinically marginal." If asked, I might have said that this spot was a fine place for observing unobtrusively and for sketching a chart of seating patterns although it was not nearly as useful for my purpose as a seat in the back row would have been. Nevertheless, two decades in medical education had made it "more comfortable" for me to take an occasional midconference trip to the coffee urn to chart those seated behind me than to sit somewhere that suggested that I either was out of place or had no clue what that place might be.

6. *A tincture of time blurs the pattern.* Divisions and intragroup distinctions are sharpest at the beginning of rotations and sharpest of all in the first few months of the academic year.

As the academic cycle moved toward its end-of-June close in both of the years I kept charts, the young became bolder in their ranks. This is an appropriate and looked-for assertiveness, for if the seating pattern in a clinical conference obliges the young to know their place, the object is not to keep them in it forever. As spring approached, third-year students were no longer stark beginners; fourth-year students, the subinterns, were anticipating graduation and the beginning of their residencies. Interns were soon to be in charge; second-year residents had been running the show for what seemed to them like forever; third-year residents would soon leave for real-life practice or assume the gray coat that fellows wore as apprentice faculty members. Here and there, beginning in late April and generalized by the end of May, decisions about where to sit at firm conference were made by the younger participants with more freedom than earlier in the year. Students took chairs next to residents uninvited; there was more mixture within ranks.

The sudden absence of students in the middle of June in both years was a shock to the proceedings. Students seldom speak in hospital conferences. Fourth-year subinterns and even a third-year clerk might occasionally present a case, especially late in a rotation—and "late" occurs earlier and more frequently as a year goes on. There is no overt reason students may not ask a question, and on rare occasions they did. Now and then they might be asked one.[15] But, for the most part, throughout the year they are silent but reliably ubiquitous observers. Their status as learners underwrites the pedagogical process in ways that residents, who, after all, are also working physicians, no longer are quite able to do. When the students disappeared in early June, having completed their work three weeks before the end of the clinical year, it was as if the glue had dissolved from the conferences. Some sessions became too pleasantly casual; some drifted a little aimlessly; the tendency was to reach the diagnosis too quickly. The second year, conferences in the last week of

June were canceled. The new clinical year brought new learners into every rank—students, residents, fellows, junior faculty—and the ritual was restored early in July.

Hierarchy, Responsibilty, and Self-Knowledge

These observations are very narrow, particular, and local ones. They concern a single aspect of professional behavior in academic internal medicine in two North American teaching hospitals. Although visiting physicians and fourth-year students—the dozen or so who were recognizable to me over 18 months—had no trouble choosing a seat appropriate to their status, no claim is made for the generalizability of these findings to other institutions or to difference spaces. Studies at other institutions might very well challenge and surely would refine these observations. An investigation of patterns of oral interaction, whether volunteered, invited, or compelled—"When to Speak at Firm Conference" paralleling "Where to Sit"—would produce a fuller description of behavior in the medical hierarchy.[16] The findings for this one fairly typical service, nevertheless, are clear. A sense of hierarchy determines behavior; in clinical medicine, hierarchy *is* behavior.

Medical education, especially in the clinical years, is not just the acquisition of facts and skills. As part of the profession's implicit moral education, rituals inculcate and enforce attitudes and behavior central to good practice. Knowledge, even extensive scientific knowledge, is insufficient to constitute medicine as a profession or to certify an individual as a clinician. More telling is the physician's awareness of the uses and limitation of that knowledge and a willingness to demonstrate responsibility for its exercise. About the formation and encouragement of this awareness—a critical aspect of clinical judgment—and how it may be improved, too little is known.

Clinical education cultivates sound judgment through the slow accretion of experience and skill and the gradual assumption of professional duties, habits, and responsibility. Learning takes place in an evolutionary hierarchy, and progress is measured against an expectation of advancing roles and status.[17] The seemingly inconsequential act of choosing a seat at a hospital conference, like the rest of medicine's covert curriculum[18]—and much of its overt clinical curriculum as well—involves the display of behavior characteristic of a competent medical team player, a person of good clinical judgment. Since such competence can be only glimpsed in beginners, the next best sign is self-conscious behavior that indicates the potential for developing that competence.[19] This potential is signaled in a fine balance between the assertion of one's ability and the recognition of its limits. The beginner at each of the hierarchy's many stages hopes to avoid either the embarrassment of looking and sounding stupid or unprepared or, ultimately worse, the hubris of claiming more knowledge or competence than can be sustained in practice.

Those who possess clinical knowledge and expertise array themselves visibly, recognizably at every hospital conference. On entering a communal room in a hospital every physician must present himself or herself as a person of trustworthy judgment, ready to sit up front and take responsibility. And, until the real thing comes along, the young must indicate that they possess a readiness appropriate to their rank, neither reluctant nor too eager, to acquire that competence. The unspoken seating rules offer a test of every attendee's self-assessment of clinical competence, and hospital conferences provide a regular, evolving opportunity for its symbolic display.

PART IV

Clinical Judgment and
the Nature of Medicine

CHAPTER TEN

◡◠

The Self in Medicine: The Use
and Misuse of the Science Claim

Men plug the dikes of their needed beliefs
with whatever mud they can find.

—CLIFFORD GEERTZ

ONCE AT A Modern Language Association conference, an English professor in
his midthirties introduced himself to me just as a session was about to begin.
He said a little urgently that he'd like to talk afterward. He'd be going the
next year to a well-known medical school.

"That's great," I said. "Congratulations!"

It was welcome news. The school he named had long had a medical ethics
program but had never hired anyone in literature or any of the other medical
humanities. About time! I looked forward to the conversation.

But as it turned out, he hadn't been offered a job. He'd been accepted as
a student. He was set on going, but uppermost in his mind was a question.

"Is it going to change me?"

The question haunts younger people going straight from college to medical
school, and it's a serious question no matter who asks. Here was a chance to
talk about what I was learning about the oddities of clinical judgment in a field
dominated by science, including the fact, startling to a teacher, that character
is both crucially important and given no overt attention. Instead, still a little
disoriented (and disappointed, I confess), I blurted out the obvious answer.

"Sure! It's going to turn you into a doctor."

That, of course, was just what concerned him. What does becoming a
physician do to the person who becomes one? Plenty, I knew. But how to

describe it? Part of the difficulty is that I can't entirely know the answer because I'm not a physician. I didn't go through the arduous preparation in biology and the long clinical apprenticeship. But no physician I've ever asked can quite describe what it does either. The self that attempts the description is the new, acculturated self, one who takes for granted some of the most profound changes.[1] A set of pre- and post-tests might provide an answer, but the most important qualities—ways of looking at the world, ways of *being* in the world, aspects of the self the English professor worried medical school might change—are more difficult to capture. In tackling that larger question, this chapter, even more than most, must be an essay, a trial account of the part medicine's claim to be a science plays in the process of turning science students (including those who once were English professors) into physicians.

Two things—besides their professional knowledge and skill—set physicians apart from the rest of us, two things that shape them as people: a familiarity with death and an odd relationship to science. The two are not unconnected. Death is always present but is seldom discussed in medical education.[2] In the first year, students dissect human bodies with knives, scissors, saws, fingers. Then, after a two-year barrage of lectures, they begin to learn the practice of medicine in tertiary-care hospitals where, especially since the late 1980s, almost every patient is seriously ill. By their third year (and as early as the second in some schools) students regularly encounter gravely ill people for whom time is running out. They question them about intimate details of their declining lives; they examine their failing bodies.

Much can be done to postpone dying, but it cannot be prevented. When patients' deaths are imminent and when they die, students are there. Later when students become residents, they are responsible for diagnosing fatal illnesses, treating patients close to death, fending it off, and finally pronouncing it. Even though death is sometimes welcomed, occasionally encouraged, for most physicians it remains the great enemy. Some students choose psychiatry or one of the "cheerful" specialties like obstetrics or pediatrics, but while the patients of those specialists very seldom die, it is all the more cruel when it happens. Besides, by the time new physicians enter residency, in a personal sense it is too late. By then the cadaver has long been dissected and two years have been spent rotating through hospital wards where death is a constant presence. Thus, even before residency begins, every medical school graduate is well acquainted with most of the random misfortunes of human existence and far too many of the intentional evils.

Against this onslaught, young physicians have their budding clinical skills and the profession's goal of exercising a cool, rigorous, scientifically informed rationality for the good of the patient. They have not become scientists, not by going to medical school and completing a residency, but they have acquired crucial intellectual and behavioral skills and a rational clinical method. They have absorbed a commitment to objectivity: close observation, the suspension of judgment until information is gathered, skepticism about information they have not acquired or witnessed themselves, and, when results don't make sense, skepticism about their own procedures. They have learned a careful, rational method that enables them to sort through what once were bewildering signs and symptoms and now make medical sense of them. As they gain a capacity for clinical reasoning, they can begin to diagnose and treat an array of diseases with a fair degree of reliability. Their commitment to objectivity and their mastery of clinical method, both essential to clinical reasoning, enable them to do what is best for the sick people whose care is their responsibility. This is not science but clinical judgment. It is the exercise of phronesis, the situational reasoning necessary in practical endeavors. It is not just the possession of information or the ability to infer it from circumstances (although both are important) but the practical ability to select the right pieces of that knowledge for determining the best course of action in a given case.[3]

"Science" is not a synonym for rationality. Yet one can see that physicians' rational procedures, often hard-won in the face of patients' need and exercised in a biological framework, could easily come to be labeled "science." With its commitment to objectivity and thoroughness, clinical reasoning produces what certainty is possible in the uncertain undertaking of clinical medicine. It enables physicians to ignore torn and distorted bodies, awful sights, nauseating smells, the patient's misery and pain, and the promise of worse to come in order to do what must be done to ameliorate—often repair or cure—such conditions. By this circuitous route, the claim that medicine is a science comes to sustain physicians in the face of uncertainty, helplessness, and death.

The Ethos of Medicine

Emile Durkheim observed that each profession has its own morality, and medicine is no exception.[4] Aristotle's *Nicomachean Ethics* explains how it works. Phronesis or practical reason is one of the characteristics of the virtuous person, even the central operational one: you must be a good person to possess practical reason, and, conversely, the habit of phronesis will promote virtue in the practitioner. So entwined are ethics and practice that it is not surprising that they seem to be one and the same. The values of clinical practice include attention to the patient, reliance on one's own perceptions, awareness of one's skills and their limits, careful observation, thoroughness, and accurate representation of what has been seen and done. Because these values are held to be essential to good patient care, they are identified with clinical goals and obscured as moral virtues possessed by individuals. Students absorb these clinical values, and residents are judged by them without their ever becoming the subject of a class. Even in medical ethics courses, as elsewhere in the curriculum, they are basic assumptions. And while clinical medicine shares some of its values with science, the overlap between the two is far from constituting an identity.

For indirect evidence that the moral is buried in the clinical, there is the casual narrative formula that often introduces an informal case presentation. "This patient walks in . . ." a physician will begin. "Walks in" is a more vivid variant of "comes in," and both phrases are markers of an account of real-life experience. The listener is about to hear about a new or unusual phenomenon, the confirmation of old truths, or, as the speaker might label it, an "interesting case."[5] The present-tense verb suggests a more recent event than the distant, "We had a patient . . ." or "There was this one guy . . ." I puzzled over "walks in" for several years, noticing its persistence and its use by physicians at institutions other than my own. As a narrative device, the words are innocuous enough. "This woman walks in . . ." suggests that what follows will be a personal rather than a professional anecdote. ("True story!" as physicians are likely, parenthetically, to declare.) Unless spoken by an emergency physician, the words usually signify that the source is the narrator's office practice rather than the hospital. As the audience, we are taken back to that moment of clinical beginning when nothing is known and almost anything can happen. "This elderly man walks in . . ." and with the physician-narrator we are once more on the spot, curious and a little wary: What is going on here?

The moment is central to the ethos of medicine, to its identity as a profession. The physician's responsibility is to figure out what the matter is and what will be best to do for the patient. The patient must be greeted, the history taken, a physical examination performed, and at least a tentative diagnosis given. Tests may be ordered, a prescription written, a prognosis essayed. The physician-teller, responsible in the story for what was said and done to the patient, is now responsible for its accurate representation. But here's a puzzling thing. Physicians in the United States scarcely ever see a patient walk in. They don't, except by accident, see patients enter an examination room, and they almost never see anyone enter the reception area of the outer office. The alternative "comes in" elides this fact while doing all the work of marking the patient's presentation. "Comes in" is self-evident: after all, there the patient is. "Walks in" is used despite being almost certainly the one "fact" about the patient's presentation that the physician has not personally observed.

The phrase is all the more interesting for that. If "walks in" is not part of the "true story," it must serve some other purpose. A phrase used repeatedly is not accidental, and to say that its use is a narrative convention begs the question. The phrase rings true, I believe, despite the physician-narrator's literal ignorance of the patient's literal walking in, because it emphasizes the fundamental situatedness of medical care. "Walks in" suggests the patient's voluntary arrival and submission to medical attention. It designates the starting point of all clinical knowing and underlines the attention that the practice of medicine requires. It evokes the potential surprise of clinical practice, the daily presentation of the unexpected and the as-yet-unknown, and reminds listener (and teller) of the complexity and the contingency of the clinical task ahead. It marks the physician's existential situation. Here is someone in need asking for help and a second person asking what the trouble is, what he or she can do. The power of beginning with "the patient walks in"—that is, the truth of the phrase—lies in its representation of both the physician's intellectual task and the profession's moral duty.

"The patient walks in" is a Levinasian moment. Emmanuel Levinas, the Lithuanian-French Jewish philosopher, held that before knowing, even before consciousness of being, human beings are confronted with the ethical.[6] We are face to face with another whom we are compelled to recognize and acknowledge. We are constituted as persons, he believed, by our response to that other. It is our ethical duty and it precedes our own existence. Here is a post-Heideggerian philosophy very well suited to a service profession, and it bears an elemental truth for physicians. A physician becomes a physician only by taking care of patients. Medical education confers a social identity and a way of looking at the world that lasts beyond a clinical career, but a physician without a patient is not a clinician any more than a sick person without medical attention is a patient. Levinas captures this dyadic relationship. The patient's presentation to medical attention is just such an *en face* encounter. It is the moral claim at the heart of the medical encounter.

This inseparability of the moral from the diagnostic and therapeutic in clinical medicine is the germ of the clinical imperative, the demand physicians make of themselves to identify, treat, and (if at all possible) cure each patient's malady. Not that individual physicians—or whole segments of the profession—at times do not fail in their duty, but such failures are always shocking. Alice Walker's story "Strong Horse Tea" turns on a white doctor's refusal to care for a seriously ill black child. Even the doctor, it tells us—*even the doctor*—who has a duty that transcends politics and the biases of society, was casually evil. So, too, the worst of the Holocaust is represented by concentration camp experiments conducted by Nazi physicians. And the physician who certified, despite the evidence, that the antiapartheid activist Stephen Biko was faking brain injury and able to endure more "interrogation" came to represent the worst evils of the South African regime. The letter of apology that physician wrote years later acknowledges this: "I failed in my duty toward Mr. Biko in accepting certain information as given facts and making assumptions about important aspects relating to Mr. Biko's condition, without having made proper inquires or investigations thereafter. . . . [I]n failing and neglecting to examine Mr. Biko thoroughly and adequately, I was the author of my own misfortune."[7]

Such acts violate the primary duty of the profession, to recognize and care for the person who enters a doctor's office or hospital asking for help. The obligation carries over into professional life as a whole, requiring behavior, including adherence to moral and cultural norms that might seem to have little to do with professional skill: such things as promptness and deference to one's elders described by Charles Bosk or, as chapter 9 argues, something so apparently trivial as choosing an appropriate place to sit at a hospital conference.[8] Professional ideals merge readily with the ritual markers of those ideals.

If I wax a bit eloquent about medicine's ethos, it is because I believe that when all goes well, the doctor-patient relationship is one of the triumphs of human society. In every culture, medical practice is an ameliorating activity designed to salve some of the common and most grievous ills of the human condition. Its failure is not the inability to achieve a cure but the failure to attend to the plight of the sick or injured person, and it is a painful violation of trust. It takes its place on a scale with a parent's desertion or a teacher's seduction. For sentimentality I'm not a patch on the Spanish psychiatrist, Pedro Laín Entralgo, who traces a quasi-sacramental relationship back to the Greeks or the French, who, as Michel Foucault noted, use the eroticized phrase, "le couple malade," for the relationship.[9] The relationship is powerful. It underwrites the old truism that the physician's best clinical instrument— diagnostic or therapeutic—is the physician herself.

How in the world is that capacity acquired?

Culture and the Self

"Osmosis" is a term that is often used for clinical medicine's educational process: the diffusion of a solvent into a solution through a semipermeable membrane. The metaphor is a good one. The solution undergoes slow change molecule by molecule, and there's no going back. Despite all those science classes, the quintessential lessons in how to practice medicine are learned by immersion, absorption. And beyond the decision to go to medical school, students do not choose the lessons. This transfer of agency is reflected in the words the medicine-bound English professor and I used. He was not the subject but the object of our verbs: "Will it change me?" "It will make you a doctor." Medical education, especially initiation into the culture of medical practice, is the agent. He was not compelled to go to medical school or to choose a new vocation. But, having chosen, he would not be in control of its operation or its principal effects.

No one in these days of ethnic consciousness believes that culture and individual psychology are entirely separate. Nor is this awareness new. Karl Marx, in the "Eighteenth Brumaire of Louis Bonaparte," wrote that human beings make their own history, "but they do not make it as they please; they do not make it under self-selected circumstances, but under circumstances existing already, given and transmitted from the past."[10] John Dewey's exploration of the relation of character and morality in *Human Nature and Conduct* identifies "habit" as their point of confluence; it affects both individual will and social function. "The social environment," he wrote, "acts through native impulses and speech[,] and moral habitudes manifest themselves."[11] After Dewey, the relation of culture and the self endured decades of neglect at the hands of behaviorists in psychology and their counterparts in anthropology. Since the late 1970s, however, the relation of culture and the self has been increasingly well studied in the social sciences. First in Europe and then in the United States, sociologists, especially those influenced by Anthony Giddens, have focused on the interaction of self and culture. The question, writ large, is one that also engages literary theorists and historiographers: Is behavior the result of individual choice or cultural predetermination?[12] Looked at closely, as it must be, the question complicates itself: To what degree is individual choice shaped—or compelled or restricted—by culture? Beyond that, how is cultural predetermination shaped by individual choice, one's own or those of one's predecessors? How do the two interact?

The work of the sociologist Pierre Bourdieu furthers Dewey's argument. In reflecting on his ethnographic studies of both the Kabyla of North Africa and his own kin in the mountainous Bearn region of southwest France, Bourdieu moves each half of the interaction of culture and psychology into the territory of the other. For him they meet in *habitus*, the individual's cultural predisposition to perceive or know or act. *Habitus* informs an individual's learned but unreflective practices, practices that are not only shaped by culture but shape and perpetuate it, too. It is an ingrained orientation that reinforces what can and cannot be thought in the culture. It thus, according to Bourdieu, is "the engine of social stability and psychic cohesion, individual identity; a subtle probability calculus that invokes a knowable future for members of the culture." Inherited and absorbed, *habitus* is a culture's "embodied history, internalized as second nature and so forgotten as history"; as such it "gives practices their relative autonomy" and their "retrospective necessity." This self-reinforcing "forgetting" is the subject of one of Bourdieu's most interesting observations, quoted in chapter 8, that a practice "exclude[s] from the experience any inquiry as to its own conditions of possibility." The possessors of *habitus*, he points out, tend to reject details "capable of calling into question its accumulated information." This "nonconscious, unwilled avoidance" leads him to conclude that "the truth of practice [is] a blindness to its own truth."[13]

Bourdieu might have been describing clinical judgment. Such individually embedded cultural automatism is, in fact, just what clinical education aims for: an ingrained capacity for assessing the best information at hand and acting as others educated in the same culture or profession would—or at least in ways those others would recognize and accept. His concept of *habitus* is practical reasoning or phronesis understood in its cultural context; it is a kind of knowing or embedded tact that some might label intuition. Like Sherlock Holmes's "deductions," it is often astonishing to outside observers, but within its culture, such knowledge seems "natural" and "automatic." Like clinical judgment, *habitus* erases itself and becomes invisible. Those who possess it take it for granted. Like people who are experienced drivers, they "just know." What they "see" and how they respond are as plain as the nose on their face. They simply do what has to be done, what "anyone" would do.

In this, Bourdieu's *habitus* bears a resemblance to common sense as Clifford Geertz has described it, as an encoded but interpretable "cultural system."[14] Clinicians will declare that not much of their day is spent on science. To someone who knows relatively little about the workings of the body, this seems absurd. "Five percent, tops," I've heard oncologists (of all people!) say dismissively. The rest of their mental activity, they maintain, is just "common sense." Now common sense, as Geertz points out, is uncommonly complicated. Contrary to its implicit claim, it is not common at all. It is not the unmediated apprehension of reality or a grasp of the matter-of-fact, available-to-all-comers meaning of experience. Instead, Geertz says, it is a "relatively organized body of considered thought," "a cultural system," that, while varying in content from culture to culture, characteristically denies in every culture that it is interpretive at all. "As a frame for thought, and a species of it, common sense is as totalizing and dogmatic as any other"; only the stylistic features, marks of attitude, and shadings of tone ("of course") of these "frames for thought," he believes, are cross-cultural.

So it is in medicine. What counts clinically is the ability to sort through incomplete and potentially imprecise information to determine what is going on with a particular patient and then, often without much in the way of certainty, to choose an effective course of action. This may come to seem like common sense, but, if so, it is common sense about very uncommon matters. Its givenness is based on years spent studying biology and more years of hospital apprenticeship with examination piled on examination well into the physician's late twenties and thirties, long after college classmates have been made partners, started businesses, begun families. It is "common" only to others in medicine and then often only to members of the same subspecialty. Wherever common sense occurs, according to Geertz, it appears to be "natural, practical, thin, immethodical, proverbial, accessible," all qualities that "are bestowed by common sense on things, not bestowed by them on it" (88). Clinical medicine operates as if it were a commonsense cultural system, and the aim of medical education is to make it so. Medicine is an acquired rationality that is culturally engendered, communally reinforced, interpretive, situationally sensitive, and therefore dialogic and aphoristic in character—even if, as in solo practice, the dialogue is internal and the proverbs are uttered silently.

Common sense, *habitus,* phronesis, clinical judgment: there are distinctions among these concepts, especially in the degree to which they are regarded as conscious and open to alteration or refinement. I have juxtaposed them not because I assume that medicine is a culture unto itself like Geertz's Balinese or Bourdieu's Kabyla or that medicine is a subculture occupying a distinct space within the larger U.S. or Western culture, interacting wholistically with it. Medicine is an integral part of that larger culture. It is bound up with it just as methods of healing and ways of addressing illness and death are in every society. When elders of the white-coated tribe utter proverbial wisdom or focus the attention of the medical young on clinical skills, habits, beliefs, and customs, thereby turning them into physicians, they do so on our behalf. Our cultural beliefs and the assumptions we make about medicine authorize their clinical practice and the rituals of medical education, including its worst, mind-numbing, spirit-deflating aspects. The self-altering changes a medical student undergoes in becoming a physician are minor tremors compared to the tectonic shifts required to alter that process of acculturation.[15]

Bourdieu's habitus and Geertz's common sense are useful concepts because, like Aristotle's phronesis, they characterize a kind of knowing that is not hypothetico-deductive, not scientific, but nevertheless deserves the label "rational." Those who possess this rational capacity or virtue in great measure are often regarded as wise. Yet, as the philosopher Charles Taylor has pointed out, rationality as a whole has come into ill repute precisely because contemporary Westerners have no standard except science for what is rational.[16] We regularly employ no other concept of rationality. Since the mid–twentieth century, a good chunk of philosophical and anthropological thought has been occupied with accounting for ways of knowing that do not fit a positivist account of science. Those interested in clinical judgment, that *je ne sais quoi* of medical practice, could read that work with profit. Because competent clinicians embody a habitual and "automatic" commonsense method of responsive knowing, the idea of a rationality that is both deeply ingrained and largely unaware of itself is essential to understanding their enculturation, the formation of the professional self.[17]

The Self in Clinical Education

Medical students have committed themselves to a self-altering course of study. An education in clinical practice is, necessarily, a moral education. It focuses on the development of good clinical judgment that will lead to the habitual good choices: the selection of the best possible action to take in uncertain circumstances.[18] Because clinical education is an initiation into a practice, it involves the whole person: attitudes, values, behavior, habits, emotions, and ideas.[19] Such a thoroughgoing process is necessary because the clinical practice for which students and residents are being prepared concerns above all how physicians act on behalf of ill people. Theirs are not abstract decisions. Novice physicians must learn how to conduct themselves and, especially, how to determine what action to take in situations of confusion, worry, crisis, disappointment, suffering, grief, deep human need, and occasional joy. And because practical reason, as Aristotle noted, is the property of the experienced rather than the young, clinical education is designed to age the new physician as rapidly as possible.

There are no classes in clinical judgment in medical school—although recent curricular reforms have made room for medical decision-making, problem-based learning and evidence-based medicine, which come close. For the most part, students are expected to acquire clinical judgment and the behavior and attitudes that are part of it during their hospital training. An awareness of the experiential grounds of good judgment probably lay behind the objections raised to teaching medical ethics 25 years ago in the United States when faculty curmudgeons declared the whole enterprise misguided. Don't people learn their morality at their mothers' knees? they objected. Won't students learn all they need from observing the practice of senior clinicians? Ethicists were not so much proposing to teach morality as offering ways of reflecting on it (and encouraging the habit of doing so), but so long as attending physicians rather than residents did most of the clinical teaching, the curmudgeons had a point. Professional values and attitudes and habits are not learned from lectures or textbooks. They are acquired experientially by students whose prior values are shaped and refined (and sometimes changed) by contact with the attitudes, habits, and values of medicine. When it comes to teaching clinical judgment—how to figure out what best to do for patients in particular situations—clinical education has been remarkably effective, and it is not surprising that experienced physicians were inclined to see this as sufficient and inseparable from ethics. Ethics courses seemed unnecessary because a moral education—learning to exercise the virtues of good medical practice—is what the clinical apprenticeship provides.

For medical students, becoming a physician involves the absorption of a culture and the shaping of the self. It is not the formation of the self, to be sure; the curmudgeons were surely right about mothers' knees. But medical education is concerned with manifestations of that self in and through the culture of clinical medicine. So compelling is this personal and psychological aspect of education that in discussions of the experiential learning that occurs in the third and fourth years of medical school and especially in residency, the word "training" is customarily used far more often than "education." Distinguished physician-educators like William L. Morgan have objected to the term. "Training" seems too mindless, too behaviorist, more a matter of the reflexes than the will.[20] But the durability of "training" in medical discourse testifies to the importance of what is taking place and the whole-person level at which it is happening. The clinical acculturation of the physician proceeds in the face of naïveté and rank ignorance, to say nothing of the tensions inherent in clinical decision-making and the possibility of a patient's death. Indeed, uncertainty and the threat of death pervade clinical education. They give the culture of medicine its texture, and they inform the student's accommodation to its practice. The claim that medicine is a science with an ideal of quantifiable certainty and unfailing replicability, a defense wielded against uncertainty and death, is a part of that culture.

Medical students and undergraduates hoping to go to medical school seem never to be told that the education they are undertaking will have as much to do with their character, judgment, and behavior as with their intellect. Once in the hospital, clinical decisions and the acts they entail are regularly judged to be "appropriate" or "inappropriate," code words in an uncertain domain for "good" and "bad." Yet little explicit attention is given to the character or the self of the person who is becoming a physician. Instead students are immersed in daily work that relies on conducting themselves responsibly, exercising good clinical judgment, and taking appropriate action on behalf of the patient. So important are objectivity and detachment believed to be for carrying out these duties that the self who is becoming a physician, almost on principle, seems to be ignored.[21]

The neglect of the self in medicine is in part due to the honored place of self-sacrifice in the ethos of medicine. Sinclair Lewis's *Arrowsmith* celebrates it and, like Howard Becker's sociological study 35 years later, *Boys in White*, the novel emphasizes the importance of scientific discovery, especially the challenge of infectious disease, the dreams of clinical glory, and the self-denial those dreams inspired.[22] Young men in the first half of the twentieth century looked forward to conquering disease personally, and in this they followed the call of Sir William Osler, the exemplar of clinical excellence who combined bedside acumen and attention to scientific progress at the turn of the last century. Osler represents many of the values central to medicine as a moral endeavor. Self-sacrifice is among them. In "A Doctor in the House," an essay on the need for balance in medical life, Raymond Curry quotes Osler's advice that young physicians return to medical school every five years for several weeks or months:

> What about the wife and babies, if you have them? *Leave them!* Heavy as are your responsibilities to those nearest and dearest, they are outweighed by the responsibilities to yourself, to the profession, and to the public. . . . Your wife will be glad to bear her share in the sacrifice you make.[23]

Osler's "yourself" is an entirely professional, male self, and he could not have imagined as a wife a physician with equivalent duties of her own.

In the last quarter century, that heroic vision of medicine has moderated, and clinical education has to some degree changed, too. Residency programs have adopted a less military model. Night-float plans that reduce hours on call have slowly become standard throughout graduate medical education. It has been decades since residents were forbidden to marry; there is even a couples' residency matching program to accommodate the desire to find positions in the same city.[24] Parental leave, at least for the mothers of newborns, is accommodated in a growing number of residency programs. But despite a new and, on the whole, healthy acceptance of the need to maintain a personal life along with a professional one, turn-of-the-millennium medicine still stresses the sacrifice of time and personal desire that is essential to putting the welfare of patients first.[25] Until the recent restriction of residents' work week to 80 hours by the Accreditation Council for Graduate Medical Education, the way to demonstrate thoroughness and dedication, one's fitness to be a physician, was simply not to leave the hospital. Surgeons may no longer boast of destroying the marriages of their residents as proof of their program's rigor and professionalism, but they have long been critical—not alone but chief among the specialties—of work restrictions. Their residents regularly violated the old rules; call schedules were viewed as minimums; dedicated residents, it was assumed, would exceed them. Before 2003, residency programs on probation for excessive work hours were often required to use time-off schedules that went beyond limiting hours to mandate such novelties as a day off once each week.

Whatever their specialty, residents are still immersed in a medical culture that puts patients' needs above the physician's. The hours spent taking care of patients, the lack of sleep, heroic expectations about the amount and the speed of work, multitasking, thinking on one's feet despite sleeplessness—all this is not simply hazing. A week or two, as the physician-educator Jules Cohen once remarked, would be enough for that. Deprivation and cruelty, both subtle and overt, produce alterations in apprentice physicians' behavior and self-knowledge. Yet all through the rest of their lives, they will know they can wake from sleep and respond rationally, appropriately, to another person's—even an unknown person's—need.[26] Such responsibility becomes inalienable, even if groused about and avoided. Physicians will respond; they are responsible. It is the ethos of medicine. Like the capacity for clinical reasoning, which this obligation reinforces and sets into practice, responsibility is communally acquired and shared. Along with their knowledge and experience, it is an aspect of the self they have assumed.

Science and the Formation of the Physician

Medicine's claim to be a science plays an important part in the moral education of the physician. George Engel described attention to the psychosocial aspects of illness as "the science of the art of medicine," and Alvan Feinstein labeled clinical epidemiology medicine's "new basic science"—and neither for purely rhetorical reasons.[27] Students and residents routinely hear about "the science of medicine" even as they learn a practice that is guided in ways that, though rational, are clearly not scientific. They do not seem to be disturbed by this. The role of case narrative, the use of proverbs and contradictory maxims, and ritual behavior that requires the self-assessment of one's ability are all ignored. There are too many vitally important things to be done, and the practical, flexible reasoning they are acquiring is essential to performing those tasks well. Far from challenging the science claim, the educational focus on acquiring accurate information and exercising good judgment seems just what is meant by "the science of medicine"—even though that judgment is readily acknowledged to be exercised imprecisely under conditions of uncertainty.

This odd state of affairs is made possible by the fact that in clinical education the ideal of science often stands in for the intellectual and moral ideals of medicine. Qualities and habits that are necessary clinical virtues are attributed to science, even though they belong equally to medicine as a practice. Most of them, in fact, are just as important to social sciences and the humanities. Physicians will often point to the logical elimination of the possibilities in the differential diagnosis as proof of medicine's scientific status, but, as I have argued, this is a fairly simple task for anyone who has the relevant information; it does not capture the real skill of clinical reasoning. Physicians' commitment to objectivity and rigorous clinical method is a more persuasive example. Their careful, thorough, rational method may be shared with science, but an ideal of clear-eyed observation and careful reasoning is just as important to good practice in fields like history or anthropology that must explain unique circumstances and anomalous cases and contend with potential subjectivity. Likewise, the regular communal review of the detailed steps of clinical knowing in teaching rounds and case conferences can be seen as a sign of the scientific;[28] and case narrative that all but effaces its narrator reinforces a sense of objectivity. But case review is a requirement of knowing in practice, and, as I have shown, case narrative is less the proof than the condition of the clinician's objectivity, a condition shared with the law. Physicians' demand for firsthand information in clinical practice also is regarded as characteristic of a science. Clinicians will scarcely utter an opinion without having examined the patient themselves, and they prefer that tests be performed in familiar laboratories. This is not snobbery or a quest for profit (although it can promote them) but a requirement of knowing in practice. Clinicians know their frailties and trust their strengths. Their drive for firsthand information is highly rational, especially in view of the experiential character of their knowledge; it is as likely to be shared with historians and literary critics, who have a similar need to immerse themselves in the record or the text, as with chemists or biologists.

Finally, the often voiced expectation that every physician, young and old, in and out of academic medicine, will keep up with research seems to be proof that medicine is a science. The expectation includes not only knowing about trials of new therapy but now, with the advent of clinical epidemiology and evidence-based medicine, keeping up with studies of the validity and reliability of signs, symptoms, diagnostic tests, prognoses, and preventive measures as well. These may seem like the activities of a science, but they are shared by academics of every kind. Physicans have a professional duty to maintain and improve their clinical judgment. Because the soundness of that judgment depends on the quality of the information they draw upon, in an ideal world it would be informed by the best available statistical evidence about every aspect of practice. This is precisely the role of evidence-based medicine strategies, which make stepwise and methodical—that is, bring to awareness—some of the reasoning that heretofore had seemed "intuitive." Evidence-based medicine informs but does not replace clinical judgment.

These characteristics—the commitment to thoroughness and rational method, attitudes of objectivity and rigor, the reporting and review of clinical decisions, a demand for firsthand information, the injunction to keep up with research combined with the use of scientific knowledge and technology—are all aspects of clinical medicine, part of a good physician's phronesiological duty. They are no more the defining characteristics of science than they are those of history or anthropology or art theory.

In clinical education the claim that medicine is a science, rather than being an accurate description of clinical work, is instead a behavioral and intellectual norm that expresses medicine's commitment to act on behalf of patients in a way that is as well reasoned and certain as humanly possible. "Medicine is a science" is a rhetorical claim that is meant to affect attitudes and habits. It is a moral appeal to do one's rational best for one's patients. Still, the replicability and certainty of scientific knowledge remain medicine's ideal (however unreachable), and attaining to the designation "scientist" has become part of the moral and intellectual education of physicians. This aspiration makes sense of the customary failure to distinguish between "scientific" as a description of much of medicine's store of knowledge and the substantive "science," which turns medical practice into something it is not. The science ideal is meant to encourage objectivity, diligence, and sacrifice in the young, including those who come to medicine in their thirties, and to shore up the spirits of experienced physicians facing the death of a patient or the inevitable fallibility of their practice. Thus medicine thrives by advancing its moral and intellectual goals as "science" while covertly accomplishing them by interpretive, narrative, discursive means.

Science and the Self: Certainty, Detachment, Safety

Beyond status and education, powerful advantages accrue to physicians from medicine's identification with science. It operates as a kind of ballast for practicing physicians as they rely on rational skill and personal virtue to meet their responsibility for another human being's continued health or survival. Science itself has an ethos, one that values rigor, openness, and objectivity. Medicine's claim to be a science appropriates those values. "Science" promises rigor of thought and procedure and a triumph over uncertainty. It is a specious triumph, deceptive for patients *and* physicians but perhaps essential as an ideal. In addition, medicine's identification with science also offers physicians an escape from emotion and the perils of subjectivity. No wonder they find sustenance, even comfort, in its aura and values.

First, there is emotional support in the intellectual assurance science offers. Unlike other fields where knowledge is uncertain, in medicine the stakes are high. The physician's duty is to attend to another human person, typically now in the United States a fairly random, heretofore unknown person, who has presented himself or herself for help. Intellectual rigor is essential, but even in the best of circumstances, no matter how careful and rational the reasoner, clinical reasoning is still inferential. Pitfalls abound. Jerome Kassirer and Richard Kopelman's *Learning Clinical Reasoning* is a catalogue of ways the rational mind can go wrong.[29] Even when bolstered by the best available evidence and the logical and statistical sophistication of clinical epidemiology and medical decision-making, it still neither deduction nor induction but abduction. The claim that this is science screens clinical reasoners from its inherent pitfalls. And if science, especially a simplistic ideal of it, is the only model for rationality in our culture, how can medicine not claim to be one?

Second, science provides physicians an easily described and defended ethical stance. The ethos of science is the open and unbiased pursuit of the truth of natural phenomena, an activity that often attempts to persuade us, its consumers, that it is value free. Two generations of historians and philosophers of science have demonstrated that it is no such thing: science is as much a product of its time and place as any other aspect of culture. It strives, nevertheless, for an admirable openness to all comers, a democracy, and an attempt to control bias. Medicine does well to share them. That physicians' knowledge is always situated and at its best reliably intersubjective does not obviate the goal of fairness or the need at times for a suspension of emotional involvement. Nevertheless, sharing some of the goals of science does not require the profession of medicine to label itself either morally neutral or intellectually objective or its practitioners to think of themselves that way.[30]

Last, for many physicians the principal benefit of the belief in medicine as a science is the boost it gives to clinical detachment, the professional façade maintained in the face of illness, pain, and human disasters of every sort, especially a patient's untimely death. Physicians practice in circumstances that (as every patient knows) are the focus of human emotions. Fear and the possibility of death, even if they are not everyday occurrences, are always at hand. Clinical detachment was physicians' interpersonal goal long before Sir William Osler gave it its best known expression in his essay, "Æquanimitas."[31] The satiric novelist Samuel Shem acknowledges this need in Law IV of *The House of God*: "The patient is the one with the disease."[32] Surgeons, likewise, are forbidden to bleed. Under such constraints and faced with all sorts of natural and accidental disasters, there is little wonder that physicians call on whatever aid they can muster. After all, how to be attentive to another human being without losing oneself is a problem every human being struggles with in one way or another: how to care for children, spouse, parents, friends without being overwhelmed. (And if we do not struggle, it may be because we have reinforced ourselves with something like the clinician's detachment.)

Physicians, new and old, need a safe way of being in contact with other human beings and their own feelings. Rita Charon has written that the "detached concern" of physicians described by Renée Fox is just that, a description, and was not meant to be a clinical goal at all; Jodi Halpern has argued that detachment impairs decision-making, while what she calls "emotional rationality" promotes better patient care.[33] Besides, the detachment supplied by the ideal of science does not deliver on its promise of protection from emotional pain—not without a cost to the physician's ability to feel. More than three decades ago, David Reiser described the carapace that forms when detachment is not balanced by engagement.[34] More recently John Lantos has written of his fellow resident's plea for a little time to mourn the death of a patient and of how little residency has changed in the years since.[35] A number of clinicians have experimented with the admission of emotion into accounts of practice: William Branch and Anthony Suchman describe the meaningful encounters that physicians report with patients and their families.[36] The long tradition of personal essays in the *JAMA*'s section "A Piece of My Mind" is now matched by "On Being a Doctor" in *Annals of Internal Medicine* and "Narrative Matters" in *Health Affairs*. The American Board of Internal Medicine's End-of-Life Patient Care Project includes, in addition to its clinical report, a companion collection of stories about caring for the dying by its clinical experts.[37] In writing about their experience, physicians can find support from philosophers, psychologists, and other clinicians who argue for the place of emotion in the rational life.[38] Emotion is not irrational. On the contrary, feelings operate as a bellwether for rational investigation—in medicine and out.

Far from providing a safe way to be in contact with patients, medicine's science claim is a frail defense against uncertainty, death, and human emotion. The belief that medicine is or should be such a science exacts a toll on the personal development of medical student and residents, the lives and psyches of physicians, the aid and comfort of patients, and the role of medicine in society. The profession's dream of an objective, stable, and certain knowledge of disease and treatment may serve to cultivate clinical virtues, but in the process it has justified a frequently brutalizing medical education and an impoverished clinical practice. Contemporary medical education is too often conducted with little overt attention to the personal gifts of students, their sense of vocation, or their suitability for a service profession, and, worse, with an outright neglect of that education's effects on their lives and spirits. By contrast, despite the long-depressed academic market for university teachers, graduate students in the sciences and humanities are more likely to have the experience of being "chosen" by trusted mentors as promising future members of their discipline than are medical students. The sense of calling with which many people enter medical school too often goes unrecognized and unencouraged, and soon I wanted to apologize to the English professor for my part in that widespread neglect. Medical students are often as reified as patients, and because they are not actually ill, there are fewer limits on the interventions they are expected to endure. They have willingly presented themselves for training, after all.

Medical practice is impoverished too. The belief that medicine is or ought to be a science casts suspicion on qualities that border the practice of medicine and make its practitioners uneasy. These are characteristics of physicians that would be regarded as virtues in other circumstances: appreciation of the individual person and the anecdotal event, recognition of a person's pain, attention to feelings, an awareness of one's own emotional life and participation in the lives of others, and knowledge of the provisional nature of much of clinical knowing. When it comes to taking care of sick people, these characteristics are often regarded as flaws. The claim that medicine is a science guards against them. It mitigates the threats they pose for the care of patients: the powerful skewing effect of the single event, an overidentification with patients, the temptation to put one's own life-interests before the needs of patients, and, worst, being frozen with indecision and unable to act. The ideal of science with its implicit reminder that medicine is objective and concerned with the perilously real serves as an all-purpose defense against these personalizing tendencies. Every clinical ritual that celebrates medicine's scientific ideal or claims evidence for a scientific stance in the procedures of its clinical rationality plugs the dike against such subjectivist threats.

Yet positivist science is the wrong warrant for physicians' authority, and their idealization of science disregards important aspects of clinical medicine. The power of the patient-physician relationship, particularly the efficacy of clinical attention, is neglected, and clinical rationality is misdescribed and undervalued. Rightly understood, evidence-based medicine promises a far better defense against the perils of clinical practice than an unexamined idealization of nineteenth-century physics. Physicians are science-using, information-sorting interpreters of timebound circumstances. Their clinical rationality molds abstractions of all sorts to the care of particular patients, and evidence-based medicine addresses this clinical imperative without claiming to be a science, not even a "new basic science."

Meanwhile, the science claim continues to take its toll on physicians. It feeds what Robert Veatch long ago described as the engineering model of the physician, one that too often impoverishes the patient-physician relationship.[39] The reification of patients that is the result deprives physicians of many of the emotional pleasures of practice. Such a detached stance can become ingrained, spilling over into the rest of the physician's life, rendering human contact difficult, and promoting a sense of self as invulnerable that makes it unthinkable for a physician to seek treatment for the most obvious physical malady or psychological distress.[40]

It would surely be better—for patients, for physicians, and for medicine as a part of society—if physicians understood medicine's practical rationality, described its strengths and limits realistically, and acknowledged the quest for unbiased, certain knowledge not as a scientific imperative but as a moral and clinical one. Surely the ideal of science is not so essential to the selfhood of the physician that it cannot be replaced. Science has mistakenly come to represent both the rationality and the ethos of medicine, the professional commitment to do one's rational best for the good of the patient. In time, these have become the beliefs that count most both for the people who are physicians and for the profession as a whole. Giving up the idea that medicine is or soon will be a science and the dream of certainty and victory over death would require an awareness of method, a recognition of personal and professional limits, and, especially, an examination of the profession's attitude toward death. But it need not in any way diminish the commitment to rationality, technology, or best evidence. On the contrary, a recognition of the nature of medicine's rationality, its phronesiology, leads straight to a lifelong commitment to professional self-awareness and self-education. Anything else would be irresponsible. Giving up the science claim would also entail a new look at medical education and a consideration of both the personal qualities it fosters, including the qualities essential to the care of the self and the care of the patient that it currently disvalues and neglects. Medical education would still turn students, even middle-aged English professors, into doctors, but it might perform that extraordinary feat more effectively and more humanely.

CHAPTER ELEVEN

✑

A Medicine of Neighbors

The neighbor . . . is an essential given, namely the primitive
human solidarity upon which our existence rests.

—EMMANUEL LEVINAS

WHAT WOULD HAPPEN if medicine disavowed the claim to be a science and
emphasized instead its character as a practice? Recognizing how physicians
actually think and work would not reduce the importance and power of
biomedical science and technological advance. The physician's moral duty
to the patient would not change, nor would the intellectual obligation to
determine the diagnosis, choose the best treatment, and provide a reliable
prognosis. But the professional's social role—at least in the United States—
might be altered. I caught a glimpse of this possibility when I discovered the
appeal that the image of a "medicine of friends" has for physicians beset by
the current (dis)organization of health care.

A Medicine of Strangers, the title Charles Rosenberg gave his history of
American hospitals, struck a nerve in academic medicine.[1] Although the book
is about the nineteenth-century origins of an institution that seems to have
been with us always, its title could serve for a contemporary account of health
care in the United States. Today "the care of strangers" is an apt description not
just of hospitals but the whole agglomeration of professional mores, economic
practice, law, and custom that makes up the nonsystem we disparage and
still take pride in. Already weakened by patients' geographic mobility and
the proliferation of subspecialties, the patient-physician relationship has been
dealt a damaging blow by managed care. Increasingly, the profession that we
appeal to in our direst need is becoming—in hospital and out—a medicine

of strangers. Little wonder that contemporary physicians locate medicine's healing authority in science rather than in its best, most authentic source, the care of patients.

The assumption that medicine is a science affects more than physicians' sense of themselves. It also limits the idea of the profession's role in society. On the positive side, the democratic openness and free access to information associated with science are qualities that support the ethical commitment to provide equitable care to all comers found in many of medicine's oaths and professional codes. But on the negative side, medicine's social role is limited by the value-free objectivity physicians (along with most of the rest of us) attribute to science. Issues of public health thus are seen as political rather than professional matters. So too are the economics and the organization of health care, even when, as in the United States, medicine has become a commodity and its egalitarian ethos weakened. Only as the clinical encounter has been turned into a brief, almost mechanical, ad hoc meeting of strangers—in other words, when the care of patients is threatened—have these issues become a concern. The lack of a stable panel of patients, exacerbated by managed care (which promised just the opposite), also means that clinical detachment is easy to maintain and so is a lack of interest in public health and even in psychosocial issues. Patients, seen hurriedly one by one, are likely to pose only diagnostic and technical rather than human or social problems. Physicians, who are educated to take pleasure in solving diagnostic puzzles, working out treatment, wielding technology, and devising cures are distracted from the social and economic components of the maladies they treat.

The advances of biomedical science and clinical medicine's goals of increased precision and efficacy have not created this narrowed vision, nor has the belief that medicine is a science by itself led physicians to view their work mechanically or estrange them from their patients. But with science the ideal, the failure of medicine as a caring profession becomes less important and its detachment from the health of the community less a betrayal of its goals. Scientific and technological successes can obscure (and may even seem a necessary trade-off for) the social failure to make those wonders available to those who cannot afford them. And the more objective and scientific medicine is believed to be, the more easily it can be commodified, detached from a caring physician, and judged by its "product," health. Malpractice suits and third-party control of medicine soon follow.

Not long after Rosenberg's book appeared, I took part in a seminar on the doctor-patient relationship at a neighboring medical school, and for a time the participants, mostly physicians, wrestled with how best to represent the ideals and goals of medicine. Troubled by the idea of "a medicine of strangers," Mark Siegler spoke of expanding an essay he and James Childress had written into a book about "a medicine of friends."[2] Although I share his concern for the way medical education and the organization of practice shape the patient-physician relationship and believe images are a subtle and powerful force, the phrase "a medicine of friends" disturbed me. It took some time to work out why. Siegler has not (yet) written that book, but this chapter is a response to what I imagine might be its argument.

A Medicine of Friends

The right metaphor for the relationship between patient and physician is a question that has interested a number of thoughtful observers of medicine. And no wonder. The relationship not only engages hopes and expectations on both sides but also—and not accidentally—implies a vision of society. Images proposed for the physician have included teacher, friend, parent, priest, advocate, engineer, carpenter, scientist, detective, plumber, mechanic.[3] In such a list, "friend" seems trustworthy and solid, although maybe a bit too simple. In its place, I propose a medicine of neighbors. Far less alienating than a medicine of scientists or technicians, it is an alternative image that is more inclusive and, I believe, finally more rewarding than a medicine of friends.

The image of the physician as friend, however, has a venerable if thin history, and arguments for it are appealing. Pedro Laín Entralgo's call for the exercise of "medical philia" is probably the best known. He begins his historical survey of the patient-physician relationship, *Doctor and Patient*, with a long quotation from Seneca:

> Why is it that I owe something more to my physician and my teacher and yet do not complete the payment of what is due to them? Because from being physician and teacher they become friends, and we are under an obligation to them, not because of their skill, which they sell, but because of their kind and friendly goodwill.[4]

The idea goes farther back than Seneca. Laín Entralgo finds its roots in the value Socrates placed on friends and, above all, in Aristotle's *Nicomachean Ethics*, where friendship, a mutual good will motivated by utility, pleasure, or virtue, is an essential part of human happiness.[5] But in adopting the Greek ideal, Laín Entralgo must ignore the class structure of slaveholding Athens, and his readers must imagine themselves rich, free men who deserve the comradeship of their physician. As a psychiatrist, he identifies medical friendship with Freudian transference, a bond that facilitates the patient's recovery (9, 159); yet for him, somewhat contradictorily, friendship retains its discriminative character. It is also the benevolence accorded an individual "because he is the individual he is" (53).

So attractive is the image of the physician as friend—and I do not mean a "friendly physician"—that many writers, without argument or explanation, assume it as the ideal form of the patient-physician relationship. This may be because, as Robert Bellah and his colleagues have observed, Americans nowadays regard friendship as a variety of the therapeutic.[6] Or it may be that friendship, freely contracted between individuals, has come to replace what we lack in the United States in the way of community. Whatever the case, contemporary advocates tend to regard the idea of the physician as friend as an overlooked but self-evident value. Edmund Pellegrino and David Thomasma see friendship as related to the medical virtue of compassion: a good physician, they say, is compassionate, like a friend, but brings a competence to the relationship not required of friends.[7] James Drane, in his Aristotelian argument for virtue ethics, goes farther: "friendliness" in his binary view is the "key virtue in medicine."[8] Likewise, Rosamond Rhodes's plea for the reconciliation of justice and care in "Love Thy Patient: Justice, Caring, and the Doctor-Patient Relationship," maintains that "a theoretical perspective (call it justice, beneficence, utility, etc.) is an inadequate grounding for ethics" and that in the patient-physician relationship, "justice . . . requires a foundation of loving friendship."[9] M. Therese Lysaught celebrates friendship as an ethical standard in her response to David Hilfiker's story of Clint, a once homeless HIV-positive man making one last attempt to break his drug addiction. She notes particularly the physician-narrator's effort to overcome "the inequalities that often serve as barriers to friendship."[10] The ideal of friendship also caps Linda Emanuel and Ezekiel Emanuel's models of the doctor-patient relationship; their "deliberative model" calls for the physician to engage in values clarification and moral persuasion as a teacher or friend.[11] Chalmers Clark and Gerrit Kimsma speak of "a special model [of friendship] in the physician-patient relationship" in instances of physician-assisted suicide although they argue more strongly for a collegial model that includes professional distance as well as intense personal involvement.[12]

The ideal of friendship can also be read back into classic works on the doctor-patient relationship. The title of Rhodes's essay is a reminder that Francis W. Peabody's often quoted wisdom can be read as an appeal for friendship: "The secret to the care of the patient is to care for the patient."[13] A visual image of the physician as friend is often located in W. Eugene Smith's widely admired 1948 *Life* magazine photographs, "Country Doctor." His pictures have become icons of the way doctoring used to be. The physician he depicts is out at all hours, no matter the weather, and comfortable among everyday objects in the kitchens and sickrooms of his patients' homes.[14]

The ideal of friendship is not exclusive to medicine. Rather than survey the obvious—advice to the clergy or philosophies of teaching—I will cite only the surprising: friendship as an ethical ideal for lawyers. In the 1976 *Yale Law Review*, Charles Fried's "The Lawyer as Friend: The Moral Foundations of the Lawyer-Client Relation" proposes friendship—focused on a goal, of course, but friendship nevertheless—as a model for the relationship between attorney and client.[15] Such arguments suggest that friendship is an ethical goal of professional relationships. Whether motivated by nostalgia for an imagined past or by longing for a rarely attained unanimity, these writers encourage us to believe that good physicians should count patients as friends and that friendship between patient and physician is a goal of medical practice.

Against Friendship

The best indication that the ideal of friendship is not a true goal of medicine is the odd fact that it is expressed primarily by those who belong to the profession in question and not by the people they serve.[16] For physicians, "a medicine of friends" is a critique of impersonal medical care and the increasing commodification of medicine. Attractive as it is as an ideal, it has real flaws as an ethical goal for medicine. It directly conflicts with medicine's ideal of openness to all in need, or if it does not, it is impractical: friendship with every patient would be emotionally exhausting, even perilous. Instead, I believe it is a compensatory rhetorical turn, a vivid way of rejecting the domination of current professional relationships by both the detachment believed to be a part of medicine's aspiration to be a science and the threat of its becoming simply a business. The image suggests what the speaker or writer finds wanting in the way things are, but as an ideal, a medicine of friends is in so little danger of being realized that no detailed description of it exists. Instead, it is a binary response to the alienation of patient and physician, as if "friend" were not only the opposite of "stranger" but, despite the wide range of human relationships, its only possible contrast.

That physicians propose "a medicine of friends" far more often than patients suggests that friendship may represent peak experiences in the lives of practitioners rather than their ordinary clinical assumption. Indeed, William Branch and Anthony Suchman, who asked internists about the most significant occasions in their professional lives, discovered they were times of crisis when physicians felt emotionally close to their patients and their families.[17] These are the valuable moments of connection in the service of other human beings. To recognize those connections and maintain the hope of experiencing moments like them in the future are laudable aims; but they seem to be consolation for patients' deaths and a bulwark against the alienation and detachment of medicine understood as a science. Such moments, important as they are, are not a standard for judging patient-physician relationships. They do not establish friendship as a professional goal.

A few scholars have called the ideal of friendship into question. Anne Hudson Jones and Edward Erde describe friendship between physician and patient as simply bad medicine. In the novels they examine—*Woman on the Edge of Time* by Marge Piercy (1977) and *It's Hard to Leave while the Music's Playing* by the physician, I. S. Cooper (1976)—they, too, find that it is the physician who idealizes friendship and not the layperson.[18] Patricia M. L. Illingworth, considering the interactions of AIDS care, argues that the friendship model violates autonomy of the patient who does not request it and diminishes the autonomy of the patient who is psychologically needy.[19] Ann Folwell Stanford and Nancy M. P. King, although they do not address the concept of friendship, express strong reservations about the related ideal of understanding the "whole patient," particularly when it licenses, for example, an otherwise well-respected physician (one who makes house calls!) to snoop in his patients' medicine cabinets.[20] Even Arthur Kleinman's more dialogic remedy for a medicine of strangers, the recommendation that physicians elicit their patients' beliefs about their illness, has been criticized by Michael Taussig as open to manipulative use.[21]

Medicine is an inherently unequal relationship, and to some degree it depends for its efficacy on that inequality. Given this, the physician's desire to know the patient may be an admirable change from regarding "those people" objectively, scientifically, as instances of disease, problems to be solved or, worse, mere "teaching material," but it nevertheless can be invasive and even coercive. It was something like this that I felt at the suggestion of "a medicine of friends." A good patient-physician relationship and a high standard of patient care requires that people who are ill not be coopted or their story alienated or appropriated by attempts to achieve something that looks or feels like friendship.

The doctor is not a friend. Or if she is, that is not who she is being when she is being my physician. She is scraping my abraded palm with a small wire brush, tweezing out the fine grit that remains, then applying iodine. She has paid no attention to my grimace or to the fact that I want out of here—not an examining room but the more neutral and nonbillable lab in the clinic of our hospital. She ignores my dawning realization that I was wildly mistaken when I said I'd rather not have a painkiller just before my class. This is not friendly! It is doctorly: she is intent on my hand, telling me what she's going to do next, keeping the small Ulysses contract we implicitly made about no analgesic, and in two or three minutes now, if I can just hold still, I will be eternally grateful and we will go back to being friends.

During that time, the physician has distanced herself, narrowing her focus to an injured, almost entirely decontextualized hand. This is a necessary distance, an essential objectification, and while it may be relatively easy to manage for a minor, accidental injury, it is far more difficult, if not impossible, for good, sustained care. If she were my doctor, could she persuade me to stop smoking? Would she take a sexual history? Would I hesitate to "bother" her with a cough I think is trivial or (more likely) bother her outside the office with things that *are* trivial? These abrogations of good medical care are the reason physicians are advised not to treat family members. Physicians, too, stand to lose a great deal by taking care of their friends.[22] How can they tell them "bad news" or turn to them for comfort when their own lives are difficult? Either friendship or the doctor-patient relationship must give way.

What Do Patients Want?

Friendship is not what patients want from their physicians. Certainly they are quick to condemn those who are discourteous and unfriendly. Fiction offers powerful examples of the suffering such physicians cause. Tolstoy's Ivan Ilych encounters in his first physician the same bland and uninflected bureaucratic façade he has prided himself on in his work as a magistrate. It is a distant, objectifying, above all *professional* regard that prompts the physician to debate the etiology of his patient's condition and licenses him to ignore the patient's burning question: "Was his case serious or not?"[23]

Contemporary illness narratives confirm the patient's need. The hundreds of pathographies that have appeared in the last three decades have been hurled into the void created by illness and its treatment.[24] They are written not only to make sense of baffling experience but to assuage suffering that is often not merely ignored by physicians but made worse by their chilling detachment. Reynolds Price, who receives his dire diagnosis in the hallway of a major academic hospital from two physicians who hurry off to their next task, observes: "Surely a doctor should be expected to share—and to offer at all appropriate hours—the skills we expect of a teacher, a fireman, a priest, a cop, the neighborhood milkman or the dog-pound manager."[25]

Despite their need for courtesy and respect, few patient-writers find it necessary or desirable that the physician be a friend. Franz Ingelfinger's tellingly mistitled essay "Arrogance," about his quest for medical attention, begins with the frustration of consulting friends and colleagues about the very type of cancer he himself studied and treated. [26] He is rescued by his son, who tells him, "You need a doctor." The one he finds is young and far less accomplished than he, but a good and assertive (not arrogant) physician. Within this patient-physician relationship, something important, indeed essential, can occur, and Ingelfinger's title suggests that it is not friendship but the authority that is a necessary part of care.

Even those few patients who seem to see their physicians as friends do not advocate friendship as a goal of their care. In his 1980 *New England Journal of Medicine* essay Norman Cousins tells of persuading his physician to release him from the hospital and treat him instead in a hotel where he can have round-the-clock access to film comedies that reduce his need for pain medication. [27] It is the physician's trust and willingness to experiment that Cousins values, not his friendship. In "The Art of Healing: In Memoriam David Protetch, MD," W. H. Auden addresses his physician as both a trusted confidant who left the poet's bad habits untouched and a fellow patient, "yourself a victim." But the poem's leitmotif is the poet's sadness and disbelief that his doctor can die, "not [my] physician, / that white-coated sage." [28] Both Cousins and Auden value their physicians' recognition of their predicament, and undoubtedly the recognition that grows into a kind of partnership can become a friendship over time, especially when the patient has a chronic illness. But friendship, if that is what it is, is an accidental reward and not a precondition or goal of the relationship. This is particularly important, since few patients are editors of a respected weekly magazine or internationally famous poets and likely to receive the same regard. Nor do these examples suggest that the equality implicit in friendship is finally desirable in the patient-physician relationship. We all may need to exercise control over the course of a long illness or in the face of life-threatening uncertainty, but we need someone to ask about our "minor vices" too.

Rather than friendship, people who are ill want their physician's committed but disinterested attention as part of ordinary, competent medical care. In times of crisis, they also need recognition of their situation and its implications. Ivan Ilych finds this not in the physicians he consults but in Gerasim, the butler's helper. The young peasant eases the sick man's pain by sitting with Ivan Ilych's legs on his shoulders; he carries out his bedpan; he alone does not lie about the gravity of his master's illness. He is the only one who mentions death. "We shall all of us die," he reassures Ivan Ilych, "so why should I grudge a little trouble?"

Patients do not want physicians to feel their pain or to circumvent their usual stark procedures lest they be incapacitated, make mistakes, or miss important signs. Anatole Broyard spoke for patients at their most desperate when he wrote of his uncommunicative surgeon:

> I see no reason or need for my doctor to love me—nor would I expect him to suffer with me. I wouldn't demand a lot of my doctor's time: I just wish he would *brood* on my situation for perhaps five minutes, that he would give me his whole mind just once, be *bonded* with me for a brief space, survey my soul as well as my flesh, to get at my illness, for each man is ill in his own way.[29]

Five minutes is a long time to see another human being steadily and whole. It is rare indeed and a lot like love, but it is not friendship.

Can we get rid of the ideal of a "medicine of friends"? Like the ideal of science, it serves a purpose. Besides the obvious part ideals play in shaping thought and guiding action, they have more subterranean uses: they may act as a counterweight to threats or to forces that, less than ideal, are nevertheless inescapable. I have argued that medicine's aspiration to be an anecdote-free exercise of objective reasoning exists in tension with its reliance on case narrative. The contempt for anecdotes in medicine, the most anecdotal of human activities, works to keep the flood of stories under control. Likewise, the profession's working assumption that drugs are targeted agents entirely distinct from placebos contradicts the bone-deep understanding of illness and therapy held by most experienced physicians, yet the healing power of the body and the placebo effect are seldom discussed or acknowledged.[30] And these examples dim by comparison with the profession's overarching claim: that medicine is itself a science—and in the grand, positivist sense of that word. Well-researched, rational medicine is a radically experimental enterprise: the clinical use of scientific information and technological knowhow on behalf of individual sick people in need of help. Physicians describe their work as a science in order to function with a modicum of intellectual and existential security in a field that at its most rational is still inescapably uncertain.

Like the ideal of science, "a medicine of friends" works as counterweight to a necessary but somehow suspect attitude or practice. The ideal of friendship is an attempt to redress medicine's necessary decontextualization of the patient. Physicians long not only to exercise their skills but also to have a safe way to be in relationship with their patients. The problem lies with the paradox of intimacy and distance that is central to the patient-physician relationship. It exists for other professions—lawyers, teachers, the clergy—but the license physicians have to touch the body and their familiarity with matters of life and death make the balance of intimacy and safety both especially difficult and especially important. Advocating a medicine of friends is at once a reminder of the rewards of service and an antidote to a mindset and habits that impoverish practice. Friendship prompts an ideational balance. For physicians to invoke a medicine of friends is to remember that the patient, recontextualized, is after all a person. Moreover, friendship does not go too far—as another translation of *philia* might—because a medicine of friends, even in that never-never land where ideals are realized, stops well short of what contemporary Westerners categorize as love. Friendship guards against, even forbids, sexual intimacy.

R$_x$: A Medicine of Neighbors

What is needed is a different image to set against the growing specter of physicians as automatons at a conveyor belt performing technologized adjustments on a succession of disordered bodies. A medicine of neighbors offers this alternative. It can provide physicians a safe way of being in intimate contact with people who are in crisis and, thus, some comfort in the doldrums of contemporary health care. Like a "medicine of friends," it enables physicians to rehumanize their practice, but it is closer than friendship to what patients want and are likely to have available to them. A medicine of neighbors offers an alternative ideal in a profession called to service, an ideal consistent with the ethos of medicine. Neighbors are people in an accidental, almost gratuitous relationship, but one no less full of possibility for all that. Neighborliness is a duty, especially in time of need, but a limited duty that leaves considerable room for both self-preservation and performance above and beyond its call. The fulfillment of neighborly duty is judged by acts rather than by motives or emotions. Distinct from love and liking, being a neighbor requires only the fundamental respect involved in one human being's recognition of another. Above all, in its randomness it is a relationship open to time, chance, difference, surprise.

As a model, a medicine of neighbors expresses much of what is valuable in the ethos of medicine, particularly its goal of disinterested service. Equally important, as financial arrangements threaten the trust patients place in physicians, the implication of a medicine of neighbors extends beyond the patient-physician dyad. Medicine is distinctive, even in a democracy, for its attention to all comers. With the decline in public education, it now may be other than the military the most nearly egalitarian U.S. institution. If their need is dire—and with the neglect of primary care it often is—people who are poor or uninsured have access to excellent medical care. Moreover, the same emergency room treats villains as well as their victims just as (once the battle is over) military physicians are expected to treat injured civilians and enemy soldiers. Prisoners, too, are supposed to be cared for. Indeed, for unfettered access to medical care in the United States, a citizen must either join the military or go to federal prison. There are exceptions to this openness, of course, but they are sources of shame. Where medicine's openness does not extend to the poor, it is because institutional policies and appointment clerks exclude them. If somehow the poor and uninsured can reach the examination room, physicians by and large will treat them.

As a part of this disinterestedness, physicians are understood to be non-judgmental. Even the old-fashioned, avuncular family doctor is imagined to be capable of attending with relative equanimity to the consequences of our weaknesses of flesh and will. Dr. Mudd lost his good name not for treating John Wilkes Booth's wound but for denying that he had seen Lincoln's assassin. These days students learn to ask "Are you sexually active? With men or women or both?" Political correctness has nothing to do with it. Physicians see this acceptance as useful for the contribution to patient care made by the information it yields. A model of the good patient-physician relationship must possess such nonjudgmental attention and retain its rewards for both parties. The physician as neighbor is such a model. It neither requires a violation of the physician's boundaries nor licenses a trespass of the patient's. It guarantees these limits even as it enables proximity.

A medicine of neighbors is a theme of William Carlos Williams's short stories, which (among many other things) are accounts of practicing between the world wars in small-town, industrial New Jersey, where he tended to immigrant factory workers. Stories like "Jean Beicke," "The Use of Force," and "A Face of Stone" are ethical morbidity-and-mortality conferences in which the narrator calls himself to account for various errors and mistakes of judgment. He fails to diagnose a child's meningitis, sees children so poor and untended that he sometimes thinks medicine is wrong to save them, loses his patience and his temper, calls children "brats," suffers bouts of xenophobia and anti-Semitism, and is never, ever unaware of class. But his patients are his neighbors and he learns from them.

Far more celebratory is John Berger's book *A Fortunate Man*, another exemplar of a medicine of neighbors. Describing his relation to his patients, the general practitioner in the north of England says he is the "requested clerk of their records," for he witnesses the births, rites of passage, marriages, losses, death that affect his townspeople.[31] He knows and keeps their secrets, and just when he thinks he cannot be surprised, he is called to treat an elderly farm wife whose complaint "down there" is unrelated (like the rest of her life) to the penis revealed on physical examination. The physician as neighbor is also at the heart of John Stone's poem "He Makes a House Call." Visiting the patient who first taught him cardiac catheterization in his fellowship year, the poet speaks of his intimate knowledge of her body (an aortic valve "that still pops and clicks / inside like a ping-pong ball") and recognizes his limited knowledge of her life: "someone named Bill I'm supposed to know." In her garden he accepts his place—"Here you are in charge / of figs, beans, tomatoes, life"—and is rewarded with a vision of his work in the larger scheme of human endeavor: "Health is whatever works / and for as long."[32]

The best patient-physician relationship, these writers suggest, is one open to learning and characterized by a little distance. Between friends, this therapeutic distance would be too likely to be abridged. A medicine of neighbors, by contrast, encourages a safe distance without authorizing wholesale detachment. "Good fences make good neighbors," Robert Frost observed, while calling attention to the forces that work against such order.[33] The image of the physician as neighbor serves as a guide for conduct equally well in a brief encounter or a long chronic illness. Unlike friendship, it does not require (in advance of the rest of late capitalist society) equality of circumstance or, a depressing thought, the reassuring sameness of ethnicity or life experience. A medicine of neighbors does not require young physicians, as a medicine of friends would, to return to the suburbs where they grew up in order to practice humanly rewarding medicine. Above all, the physician as neighbor entails a relation to community that itself is caring. Because it offers both sure footing in intimate human contact and a goal of service, it answers physicians' needs even better than either the ideal of science or a medicine of friends. Lyndon Johnson used the image in his 1965 inaugural address. Outlining his vision of the Great Society, he invoked medicine's broader mission. "In a land of healing miracles," he declared, "neighbors must not suffer and die unattended."[34] We have scarcely begun to achieve that goal.

A community of neighbors is no more a closed circle, restricted to similar people, than is the physician-patient relationship. "Who is my neighbor?" Jesus is asked by one of his disciples.[35] Whoever it turns out to be, in the New Testament parable a neighbor is that person one is supposed to "love as yourself." The answer in the story is not a friend or a member of the same tribe or ethnic group but someone from a different and despised group, the Samaritan. A neighbor is the person passing by who stops to help.

A medicine of neighbors has all the virtues of good anthropology. Like physicians, anthropologists do their work between science and subjectivity. Their field is distinctively, if not uniquely, the intellectual discipline that has struggled with the unknowability of the other and the distortions of colonialization. Their method is, first, to describe what they see as they see it and, then, to describe what they see as its participants see it. The virtues involved in this reflexive doubleness are respect, open self-presentation and tactful withdrawal when necessary. They listen attentively, ask about differences and their meaning, check their conclusions with the informant, and, above all, do not "go native," eliding the differences between observer and observed. Friendship is not a goal.[36]

Neighborliness is a virtue that has much to recommend it as a metaphor for medicine in the twenty-first century now that both science and bioethics are widely accepted. A medicine of neighbors possesses homely qualities that friendship transcends and sometimes can ignore: chief among them are a clear regard and a fundamental respect for the other. In the absence of a "content-full" moral vision,[37] these qualities are warmer and more productive than either the egalitarianism of science or a default libertarianism necessitated by cultural pluralism. More nearly minimal, less judgmental, and more circumstantial than friendship, neighborliness creates occasions for learning. It does not require self-revelation or an enduring personal bond. Instead, it calls for recognition of both the accidental character of much that befalls us and our common life, our common need, our common fate. Well realized, the patient-physician relationship may become something like friendship. Now and then, friendship is also the reward for having been a good neighbor. But neither the patient-physician relationship nor neighborliness necessarily includes it, and neither begins there. Friendship is neither a precondition nor a goal of the patient-physician relationship.

Seen as a science rather than a practice in the service of the ill, medicine easily appropriates a detachment that defends against emotion, intimacy, and death. Biomedical science focuses on altered structures and malfunctions of the body, and if medicine has the same focus, its responsibility narrows to the study of disease in laboratories and in the living containers that are patients. Although friendship may seem to be the antidote to this view, especially at a time when the social and economic organization of clinical practice has made patients strangers, the physician's responsibility is larger. Good clinical practice requires neither detachment from patients nor their adoption as friends but rather responding to them with attention and respect.

Medicine already is or should be the care of neighbors. It is a norm that was available to medicine long before clinical practice incorporated science. We are challenged now to extend the benefits of medicine not only to those we live among, our literal neighbors, but more widely to figurative neighbors with whom we share the planet. We could do worse than to imagine the physician not as a scientist or a science-using technician but as a neighbor, and to evaluate both our beliefs about medicine and the public policy to which we consent by the degree of neighborliness they permit and encourage.

CHAPTER TWELVE

⁓

Uncertainty and the Ethics of Practice

Health is whatever works
and for as long.

—JOHN STONE

ALMOST A YEAR after my daughter's diagnosis, a few months after her treatment ended, I caught a ride with a surgeon-writer from a conference in Westchester County to an exit on the Merritt Parkway where my daughter and her husband were to meet me. I'd brought with me an early version of chapter 1 for her to read, if she were willing and time allowed. Because I admired the surgeon's account of his brother's death, I asked him about the perils of writing about illness in a family.

"It's never simple," he said. "But it's your story. Hers would be very different."

What I had written was my story, I knew. When she found the suspicious lump, I had been writing about clinical judgment, the capacity for making practical decisions in uncertain circumstances. Until then I had seen the mismatch between the way medicine is taught and practiced and the claim that it is a science from a very safe distance. Her illness, I told him, had immersed me in medicine's uncertainty.

"Uncertainty in medicine is my soapbox!"

"It's not all the physicians' doing," I ventured. "Patients and their families push them to be certain." Several miles of lively conversation followed.

Then abruptly, as I remember it, he said, "Do you mind my asking your daughter's diagnosis?"

I told him everything: Stage I carcinoma of the breast, the results of all the tests, the measurements and numbers that had been stuck in my head the whole year, all the fruits of learning medicine the hard way. The DNA studies were new since he'd retired from surgery. I sketched in the treatment she'd recently finished, the unstoppable nausea, and at the end of treatment, my unexpected anxiety at waiting for normal life, whatever that might be, to begin again.

For a moment he said nothing. Then he straightened, took a new grip on the steering wheel, and began to speak. He'd been a general surgeon, he said, "and I practiced in a small town. My hospital is an academic medical center, but it's also a community hospital. People come back to us; we don't lose track of the patients we treat. I did breast surgery there for almost thirty years." He paused.

"In all those years, I lost only one patient who had Stage I disease."

All the terrifying counterarguments sprang to mind. I was ready to cite the studies of chemotherapy and HER-2/neu, the uselessness of tamoxifen for young women. I knew how partial his knowledge was. He was right about his university town and the breadth and stability of his practice, and his experience was among the best of its kind. But, however valuable, it was the experience of just one person. What about the research! The experiments! He had given up surgery before they began doing DNA tests on tumors. Beyond all those studies, there remained the researchers' summary sentence: "The severity of the disease in young women is not entirely accounted for by the known prognostic factors." How many very young women with breast cancer had he seen?

The man who not 10 minutes before had been emphatic about medicine's uncertainty and the perils of ignoring it was now telling me that my daughter would not die—or not soon, not from breast cancer. The sources of his authority were his very local knowledge, a particular and specifically embodied objectivity, and long clinical experience that responded, I realize now, to a need he saw in me. His response—the pause, the new grip on the steering wheel, his sitting up a little straighter—were all signs of his assuming a physician's answerability. There was no intellectualizing distance between him and his experience, no self-reflective gap between his knowledge and the assurance he was implicitly offering. He stood (or, in this instance, sat upright at the wheel) for the belief that my daughter would live.

The Need for Certainty

Few experiences feel as uncertain as illness. The assumption that life will go on is grounded in our bodily existence. Heel will follow toe, food will do us good, and eyes and hands and the rest of us will do our bidding. It all adds up to the everyday capacity for denial that eases most of us through most of life. In illness that assurance breaks down. We're sick. The uncertainty of it as much as pain or dysfunction, sends us to the doctor. It is this uncertainty that is relieved by a diagnosis, even a life-threatening one. Remedies take time to work, and, afterward, more time may pass before we feel "ourselves" again. For all that time the sense of control in our lives is diminished. Uncertainty, loss of control, and the damage to the sense of self are a part of illness, and, unscientific though these concerns are, we hope our physician will address them.[1]

We want cures, of course, and very often we get them. But not always, and certainly not forever. It's not news that we are mortal. But surely, this time—in our case!—it will be different. Hope feeds on the assumption that medicine is a science, and that assumption is fed in return by need. When we are ill, the power imbalance between doctor and patient, much noted by critics of medicine, becomes a desirable difference, one we hope to enlist on our behalf. The sicker and more uncertain we feel, the greater we hope that that differential is. We need medicine to be reliable and predictable and physicians to be agents of accumulated scientific knowhow. Although sick people and their families are fully capable of distinguishing between a physician's effort and its outcome, we nevertheless pin our hopes on a perfect result. We know technical skill varies from physician to physician, but we still expect them all to possess scientific information whose application will restore health and function. This expectation of a perfect outcome is contagious. Physicians find it hard to resist, too, since they have been trained to expect of themselves a perfection of effort. People with chronic diseases know better. But the well and the newly ill (and their families with them) hold fast to a misunderstanding of physicians' capacity. They'll be able to fix it. Medicine works miracles, doesn't it?

In the face of such need, physicians understandably may not explain (and may not remember themselves) that medicine, however scientific it may be, is not itself a science. There are at least two good reasons—besides lack of time—for this. First are habits of thought, both social and professional. The brilliant success of biomedicine and medical technology has come to be taken for granted in Western culture. Physicians know an immense amount about the body and have access to therapies that offer real help and often cure. All of us have come to expect an endless series of advances that have made diagnosis, treatment, and prognosis more and more reliable. At the same time, medicine is a deeply habitual practice that may rigorously review its methods and results but does not question the status of its knowledge. Its practitioners do not often think about its radical uncertainty. They ignore the rational procedures they share with practical reasoners in other professions and the conditions their method shares with inquiry in the social sciences and the humanities.

A second reason for silence is the clinical usefulness of the assumption that medicine is a science. Although wise physicians know their practice is often imprecise and always a matter of what will probably work best, they are reluctant to burden the patient with this. As patients we may not be interested. In fact, we may positively want not to know. We want physicians to diagnose and treat with confidence, and in a culture that understands the word "scientific" as a synonym for "rational," the belief that medicine is a science adds to physicians' authority and assuages the patient's fear. It may provide hope, perhaps promote healing. So, while individual physicians may never actually declare that medicine is a science, few explain that it is not. Besides, if "science" has come to stand for "rationality," medicine surely has earned the label. Physicians strive to be as rational as possible, and clinical epidemiology and evidence-based medicine have raised the bar substantially by calling to their attention the quality of information used in clinical thinking. What's more, clinical method often feels like science. Physicians observe, generate and test hypotheses, eliminate the illogical and ill fitting, and verify what they can. This reminds them of the science they learned as undergraduates. Never mind that the social sciences and the humanities work in much the same way. Or that clinical reasoning is always contextual, necessarily interpretive, and thus always to some degree provisional or that it is organized and categorized as narrative, taught with aphorisms, and tested by unwritten rules that reinforce the hierarchy of expertise. What is most apparent is the enormous improvement in the treatment of disease and injury since the introduction of science into medicine, and successful treatment is, of course, what people who are sick or injured and their physicians care about most.[2] We want the certainty of science, its authority and protection, the promise of a better future, restored health. We want its reassurance. Instead, all too often, what we get is statistics.

The Numbers

Inside the hospital, "the numbers" means test results. "Give me the numbers" is a request for laboratory values that nail down the facts. There the term seems ordinary, a guarantee of medicine's scientific rationality. But, out on the street, "the numbers" has another life, one with a history: first a long use in illegal lotteries for the numinous objects of hope and desire; then a cleaned-up nightly presence on local television once the states took over the market in all-but-impossible dreams. In medicine, too, the numbers can be a snare and a delusion. In diagnosis and treatment, test results have something like symbolic weight. They are located on a scale established by scientific and statistical studies where they mean a great deal, but almost never in isolation and seldom precisely. There is an irony to this. Ian Lawson suggested 30 years ago that in medicine, an ill person's uniqueness is expressed, oddly enough, in numbers rather than in words; the words evoked by disease and loss or recovery are startlingly common, while test results, even for people with the same diagnosis, can vary wildly.[3]

For prognosis, especially, the numbers are at best a quantified uncertainty.[4] Like Tolstoy's Ivan Ilych, patients want most to know whether their case is serious or not. What part should numbers play in the answer to that question? Sick people facing prolonged therapy need reassurance, especially when the treatment will be painful, life-threatening, or toxic in itself. Most reassuring would be the simple news that the illness is self-limiting: the sick person will soon be well and restored to normal life. But in the absence of that assurance, many patients and their families pin their hopes, as our culture has taught us to do, on science. Without control of our fate, we look for cognitive control. Gathering information about disease and its possible treatment—intellectualizing—is one way of attempting to keep hold of a sense of predictability in the world. If the body eludes our control, at least we can understand how it has gone awry and how best to restore normality. Physicians no longer flatly discourage this or perceive it as a patient's lack of trust. On the contrary: Marcus Conant, who takes care of challengingly well-informed AIDS patients, maintains: "That is the way it should be, and particularly when you cannot, in fact, save their lives."[5] Detailed biomedical information can be practically useful to patients. When treatment options are evenly weighted or when a permanent loss will be the consequence of disease or treatment, every scrap of data helps in making decisions. In addition, information makes sense of tests, justifies therapy—especially hedged bets like adjuvant chemotherapy—and restores a sense of choice that can ease the anxiety of having a potentially fatal disease. Information can also offer hope, sustaining patients through bad times. No wonder some patients want the most minute detail.

Nevertheless, scientific information is only part of what patients need. Data must be interpreted, evidence pieced together, and information sorted for its relevance to one particular patient. This is what physicians do—and why they are not likely to be replaced by computers. Just as most physicians have found a wide middle ground between lying and "truth-dumping" when they must give patients bad news, so it seems possible when discussing treatment to find a way between the stonewalling "trust me" (with a pamphlet at best) and launching into a short course in pathophysiology with a brief excursus into cell and molecular biology. The middle ground seems large enough for every physician to find a comfortable position with almost every patient. What is less clear is the part that statistical results of clinical studies should play in the answer that is offered.

Long before the Internet, statistical facts about recurrence had entered the consciousness of the average citizen without a medical degree. Five-year disease-free survival rates are part of the lore that was absorbed as scientific medicine became the folk medicine of Western culture. These days, patients know clinical studies offer the best available data on their chances of recovering from their disease, and they want to know the truth: the numbers that pertain to them and their diagnosis. It's science after all. For physicians, the beauty of statistics is that the numbers provide a scientific answer; they represent a sometimes difficult but desirable honesty. They sum up the most and best that's known about a disease and its stages. They are the best science can do. Surely the numbers should answer the patient's burning life-or-death question.

But they don't. Helpful though the facts may be for both decision-making and a sense of control, the limits of biomedical information are nowhere clearer or more painful than in the prognostic use and almost unavoidable abuse of statistics. In their need for certainty, patients ask for scientific answers. What they are given—or find on the Internet—is probabilities. Odds. The numbers are "the facts"—or their most nearly accurate representation. Yet statistics are profoundly unsatisfying. They look like the truth, but they can deceive. Even when they are accurate, they can be misleading and a source of torment.

"Does it look bad for *me*?" Statistics don't say. Survivors survive entirely; those who die are completely dead. No one survives 82%—with the grossly literal exception of amputees, and they are whole selves, wholly alive. Nor does the survival percentage predict disease-free time. It is possible that a person with a 82% chance of surviving five years without a recurrence could find the disease has returned a month and a half into the fifth year, when only 18% of her five years remains. But that would be a random occurrence; it is not what that 82% means. No matter how promising the numbers, there is no certainty that one particular patient will do well. Except in well-advanced cases when an unflinching prognosis is called for, there is no answer to the patient's question that can come close to certainty. There is no qualified negative answer, no hopeful "probably not," that is quantifiably certain. Not only do statistics fail to answer the life-or-death question patients and their families ask, the numbers make the uncertainty painfully real. Is this really the best medicine can do?

Patients and their families want more than information, something that science cannot provide. While most patients say they want more information than they presently receive, including statistics, the numbers are only a stand-in for the reassurance they need.[6] One oncologist tells her patients never to compare themselves with people who have the same disease.[7] Another says that, while he uses statistics all the time in making clinical decisions, he seldom mentions them to his patients. When, as often happens, they and their family members arrive in his office armed with print-outs hot off a web site, he suggests they not put too much stock in them, not even in information from the reliable National Institutes of Health. "You don't want to be like the man with his head in the oven and his feet in the refrigerator," he suggests. "Head was hot, feet were cold, but on average he was just fine." It's not that the numbers are *wrong*, he says, it's that they say nothing about the individual case. Not only do they not provide reassurance, the information is sometimes counterproductive. There is no certainty. If he is to provide support and honest reassurance, he must use something more than statistics.

Human beings perceive odds subjectively. In the 1970s and 1980s, Daniel Kahneman and Amos Tversky studied the psychology of risk assessment and the wide range of attitudes to risk that influence behavior, work that won the Nobel Prize in 2002. They described how the way a statement of probability is framed can influence its perception, and how common decision strategies, themselves based on probabilities, lead people to misperceive very low and very high percentages.[8] Education and experience alter this subjectivity only a little. Stephen Jay Gould could claim that, when diagnosed with abdominal mesothelioma, his familiarity with statistics saved him from seeing them as abstractions. Instead of thinking of "means and medians as hard 'realities,' and the variation that permits their calculation as a set of transient and imperfect measurements of this hidden essence," he saw them the other way around.[9] But few of us have spent, as Gould had, a lifetime quantifying biological variation. He understood that the very long right-sided tail of the survival curve for his disease—a curve with a median survival of only eight months—stood for real outliers that his own case might resemble. Not only did this realization feed his optimism, but it probably encouraged him to undertake a highly toxic experimental treatment as well. He lived almost two decades longer.

For the rest of us, physician-patients included, numbers alone are not adequate. An educated grasp of statistics, no matter how balanced and thorough, only goes part way. Sidney Bogardus and his colleagues recommend using a variety of formats—qualitative, quantitative, graphic—to communicate information about risk: words, numbers, charts.[10] This multifaceted strategy provides a useful remedy for the misperceptions apparently built into the psychology of numbers. But it does not address the patient's fundamental concern: "Am I going to die of this life-threatening disease?" There is, as

Aristotle pointed out, no science of individuals, yet this is exactly what medicine must strive to be.[11] Except at the two extremes of the statistical scale, "the numbers" cannot answer the patient's most pressing question. For most patients, if there is any hope at all, no one knows the outcome for sure.

This yawning chasm between the physician's probable facts and the patient's need for certainty is not unique to oncology. The whole of medicine is to some degree uncertain—to say nothing of the whole of life. Uncertainty haunts meteorology, aviation, cooking, and other practices that draw upon physics and chemistry, sciences with laws far more certain than those of biology. But if the fear of losing control lies behind the patient's quest for certainty, that fear can be addressed. Physicians can offer reassurance even in the direst circumstances: that they will see that the patient is well taken care of, that they will make the best possible decisions, that they will not lie. These promises are already implicit in the patient-physician relationship, but to be reminded of them when seriously ill is a comfort. Farther along, if hope for survival dims, there can be reassurances that pain will be relieved and the physician will not desert them. Such assurances do not arise only from the physicians' grasp of biomedical facts but from their fiduciary relationship with the patient. Physicians are trusted. Because the relationship between patient and physician entails attention, the exercise of clinical judgment, and fidelity, that relationship in and of itself can provide comfort and a sense of control to patients no matter how serious their disease.

There are barriers to providing such nonstatistical reassurance. In the United States, the economics of medical care and its fragmented delivery constitute two of them. But a third, more personal barrier is well within an individual physician's power to remove: the failure to acknowledge patients' questions about their fate and the temptation to avoid such topics altogether. Because the science of medicine cannot provide anything like the certainty the patient so desperately seeks, physicians—particularly those who believe they are scientists—may feel that this is not their job. And no one, no matter what they believe about their work, can enjoy feeling inadequate or ignorant or impotent. Small wonder that some physicians become routinized to the patient's need and then ignore it. They miss the opportunity to offer a different but ultimately more valuable sort of reassurance.

How best to live one's life is the central moral question for every human being, well or ill. Life-defining illness only sharpens the need for an answer. Answering such a question may not be the duty of the physician, but acknowledging its existence is only common decency, and, as an act of witness, is often beneficial in itself. Subspecialists, especially in surgical or purely diagnostic fields, are often excused from this civil expectation, but, as Patricia Benner has observed, "We must remember that [such subspecialists] are parasitic on the good physician."[12] If physicians are not to be merely technicians, it is necessary at least to recognize that the question of life's meaning lies in wait for everyone with a serious illness, and the work of medicine bears on it. This and some advice about ways to address the day-to-day aspects of life-threatening illness are part of every physician's work. That advice may be as simple as pointing out that medicine cannot do the whole work of recovery alone. Even when it cures the disease, the patient will have to work at recovering from the illness and often from its treatment. Chronic and degenerative diseases impose an equally clear duty—if only to provide printed information and the name of a patient support group. The plea of Dewitt Stettin, Jr., for ophthalmologists to offer their patients advice about adapting to life with their failing eyesight is, unfortunately, as much needed as the day he wrote it. After his macular degeneration was diagnosed, the best physicians in the country, many of them his former colleagues, said they "could do nothing more for him." His *New England Journal of Medicine* article is a damning enumeration of all the conveniences—a talking clock, the Kurzweil reader, Talking Books, dedicated radio stations—that he was left to discover on his own.[13] As long as physicians are not merely biotechnicians, it is never true that they have "nothing more to offer." Even when a patient is dying, physicians can offer honest prognoses, timely referrals to hospice care, effective pain control, and their whole presence, however brief. These are among a physician's acts of attending.

To provide the reassurance patients need, physicians must be willing to go beyond statistics, the numbers science provides. They have at their disposal not only biological and clinical facts but experience and clinical judgment, including hunches, intuition, and an experienced ear. This is wisdom of a real-life, practical kind. Some patients will ask for scientific information; many more will want statistics; but all hunger for information about the world of illness they have entered. "Is it serious, Doc?" What we all need to know, in one way or another, is how we can live with our maladies.

Whether patients and their families can give up the belief that medicine is a science is not clear. It may be as essential for us as for physicians: a kind of metaphoric goal forever unreachable but necessary to sustain us. We may need the belief in science in the same way we seem to need the surgeon's ritual reassurance "We got it all," or the internist's last-ditch pronouncement "We've done everything we can do." The need for certainty felt by patients and families undoubtedly contributes to physicians' reluctance to examine the science claim and the failure to question or counter it. But its cost is clear. When patients and the people who love them are given a life-defining diagnosis, they discover that the numbers produced by technology and central to scientific research are not enough. Though produced with something like certainty—these are the facts!—numbers alone cannot not offer the care and assurance patients need. A loss of faith in physicians and the sense that medicine has abandoned them in an essential way makes it easy to believe that medicine has become a business after all.

Medicine and the Reign of Science

What might the practice of medicine be like without its misidentification with science and scientific values? In the century since medicine added biology to its armamentarium, it has ceded its authority to science. As it has gained power from the technology that science underwrites, medicine's values have been increasingly mislocated in its outmoded ideal of scientific knowing. Medicine's identification with science is understandable. Besides improvements in diagnosis and treatment, there are its more subtle benefits: authority and emotional protection for its practitioners, an idealistic alternative to the neglect of public health and universal access, reassurance for patients. Although the idea of medicine as a science is not responsible for all the difficulties facing medicine, an examination of its effect on patients, society, and physicians themselves suggests some remedies.

A richer, more complex understanding of clinical medicine and its characteristic rationality could readily replace the flawed ideal of medicine as a science. As a moral, science-using practice whose goal is the benefit of the patient, medicine does not need the ideal of science to protect its practitioners either from subjectivity and emotionalism or from caring about their patients. The former, William Osler argued in *Æquinimitas*, can be avoided by understanding the physician's duty.[14] The latter, as Francis Peabody hoped to persuade his colleagues at the beginning of the scientific era in medicine, is in fact the key to clinical success: "The secret of caring for the patient," he wrote, "is to care for the patient."[15] Osler and Peabody are reminders that neither the idea of a patient-centered medicine nor its internal tensions are new. But a reemphasis on this wider view of medicine might wean both patients and physicians from the misplaced belief in medicine's certainty and encourage communication about risks and desires. It might dissuade physicians from self-protective but no less cruel retreats into detachment. If medicine were understood as a practice, its focus on the patient as a frame for the use of biological and clinical science would be a sufficient source for values—including thoroughness and accuracy—now attributed solely to science.

A richer understanding of clinical medicine would leave room to appreciate the clinical judgment required by the constant tensions of practice: the tug-of-war between case-based knowledge and the abhorrence of the anecdotal; the conflict between the dependence on the patient's self-reported history and the thoroughgoing skepticism about it; all the uncertainties inherent in the need for generalized knowledge to care for particular illnesses. Nor is the tension confined to methods; medicine's immediate goals are in conflict, too. The therapeutic imperative does daily battle with therapeutic nihilism, and physicians are often torn between the need to acknowledge death and the desire to do the utmost to save life.

We need to understand the practical importance the ideal of science has as a counterweight in clinical medicine's system of balances. Left unexamined, it endangers that balance. When the belief that medicine is a science dominates, upsetting the balance of information and experience in clinical medicine, it undermines and corrupts medical practice. Objectivity drives out other clinical virtues. Diagnoses are delivered in public hallways; patients with cancer are described as having "failed chemo" when chemotherapy has so clearly failed them; obstetricians forget that their 863rd delivery is the woman's first or only or last. Clinical medicine, if it is to provide good patient care, must maintain its unresolvable tensions. The quirky, unscientific aspects of clinical education—its reliance on case narrative, the subordination of the scientific idea of cause to the need to treat the patient, the use of conflicting aphorisms to guide and reinforce clinical judgment, the performative enactment of the hierarchy—all flourish precisely because they promote balance in the exercise of clinical judgment in a particular case. Science alone is a limited source of knowledge and authority in the care of patients.

The Performance of Certainty

Medicine's own authority flows from the patient-physician relationship. Although the rituals and rules of that relationship have been refined over the last 50 years, the connection between the healer and a sick human being asking for help remains central to the care of the patient.[16] Studies of performance describe how ritual idealizes its participants and events: every four years, an inauguration gives the United States a president who will do his best for the country; the marriage ceremony creates blushing, eager spouses, who are the hopeful start of a new family. Physicians participate in this ritualization of life events. Their attention to patients—their act of attending—goes a long way toward creating a therapeutic relationship. The authority of that relationship is limited, and the field of medical ethics (to say nothing of malpractice litigation) has been pointing out those limits for more than 40 years. Yet, while trust in the medical profession has declined, patients still commonly report that their own physician is different: competent, trustworthy, helpful, sometimes the source of inspiration and strength.

The performance of physicianhood is learned early, absorbed in medical school along with biological facts, clinical rules, and hospital routines. It is part of the acquisition of technique and the mastery of professional behavior and attitudes, and medical students are vividly aware of it. They put on white coats and the world responds to them differently. They often feel—as many people do when they are learning their craft—a bit fraudulent at first. Their interactions with patients slowly reassure them, alter them, and confirm them in their role. For physicians, as for happy couples and new presidents, the audience plays an important part. Patients see the person who is the physician but respond to the archetype; they evoke physicianly performance by the power of their need.

This doubleness that beginners are so aware of characterizes all performance. The drama theorist Richard Schechner, using Victor Turner's work on ritual's performative "scripts," points out that when we see a famous actor in a role—Lawrence Olivier in *Hamlet* is his example—the person we see is not Olivier but not-not-Olivier as well. And Olivier both is and is not Hamlet.[17] This is so apparent to most of us that, like Henry Fielding in *Tom Jones*, writers can depict a naive theatergoer who becomes so caught up in the action on stage that he shouts a warning to the endangered hero. The doubleness of performance is not confined to the theater. When performance takes place at an altar, on an inaugural platform, or in a doctor's office, it creates social reality. Victor Turner describes this power of ritual as "making not faking,"[18] and Claude Levi-Strauss tells of a skeptical Kwakiutl setting out to expose the trickery of shamans who slowly comes to believe in their efficacy as he himself becomes a shaman.[19] Performance confirms performers in their roles, and physicians are no exception.

The morning after my daughter's lumpectomy, a third-year medical student assigned to her case appeared in her room well before dawn.

"I've come to take your drain out," he said.

Removing a tube from an incision is not a difficult task, and she knew it. Just the day before, her surgeon had urged her to stay in the hospital overnight but added that if she really wanted to go home, he would show her husband how to remove the drain. Her husband has a degree in computer science.

But this was a medical student. All by himself. He was her age or a little younger, and before her surgery they had talked about medical school. She knew, although not from him, that it was the first week of his surgery rotation and that, because he had chosen to do the surgery clerkship early in the school year, he very probably hoped to become a surgeon.

"Do a lot of these?" she teased, knowing that if he had done any at all it would be a stroke of luck.

"All the time," he declared in a slightly ironic voice, knowing that she knew it couldn't possibly be true.

He took out the drain. She told the story.

For a long time this seemed to me a wonderful, rather wicked challenge from vulnerable patient to future surgeon, proof that her wit and sense of self were undiminished by adversity. It seemed to promise that she would survive. Irascible cancer patients have been shown to do better than mild, meek, compliant ones;[20] and this good-natured refusal to go along with the pretense that the student was a physician and she was not "teaching material" seemed feisty and admirable.

But I've come to see that it was more. She also wanted reassurance.[21] Her question was the opening line of performance, and her tone of voice was his cue. She asked the question about experience that patients long to ask, but she didn't ask it straight. She did not want the answer she already knew. Instead, she wanted to know that he knew what he was doing even if he'd never done it before. She wanted him to be confident, physicianly. His brash, equally knowing declaration would soon be true. Meanwhile, in the circumstances, it was the right answer. I think he'll be a good surgeon.

The Epistemology of Practice

The doubleness of performance suggests how the care of patients enables physicians to accommodate the claim that medicine is a science—even as the uncertainty of their practice requires much that escapes or defies the designation "science." Focusing on the patient reorients the physician's knowledge: the ethics of practice outweighs both the assumption that medicine is a science and everything the physician may understand about how clinical knowing actually works. The duty to respond to the patient, to act or to justify inaction, necessitates a sense that the information at their disposal is as solid as science. What physicians know about the uncertainty and imprecise applicability of their knowledge is one thing; the grounds upon which they respond to a patient are another. Thus the status of knowledge in clinical medicine may be uncertain, but knowledge in practice is firm. A full understanding of how doctors think—a theory of medicine's clinical rationality—can exist side by side, in the same person, with the presumption of certainty. But they are not available simultaneously. Physicians do not analyze their practice (or anyone else's) and act at the same time. Those who have worked out the uncertain status of medical knowing and its differences from positivist science nevertheless remain subject, as practitioners, to clinical medicine's ethical demands.

Medicine's moral imperative to act on the patient's behalf, we must conclude, is so strong and so thoroughly embedded in clinical habit and predisposition as to override mere ideas about their knowledge. The Levinasian face-to-face encounter with the patient, the power of one's peers, and the habits of perception and knowing ingrained by a long apprenticeship all compel the physician's clinical attention to the patient and call for the exercise of practical reason in this case. This is surely why there is relatively little interest in the status of medical knowing among physicians and almost none at all in introducing the topic into medical education. Nor, for all the reasons I have described, do patients challenge the presumption that medicine is certain and invariant. Medicine's practical epistemology, its phronesiology, may undermine its claim to be a science, but because that understanding is set aside in the care of patients, it comes to seem irrelevant. Edmund Pellegrino's intolerant dismissal of postmodernism makes sense in this context. He justifies it with the old saw, "There are no atheists in foxholes."[22] For physicians, the ethics of practice always trumps the epistemology of clinical medicine.

This trump goes far toward accounting for medicine's blindness to its own rationality and explains why so little about its actual workings is included in medical education. Such neglect otherwise makes no sense. The practical balance of scientific and experiential knowing in medicine is, after all, the overriding, if implicit, lesson of clinical education. It is the goal of every case presentation and the aim of the long, closely overseen clinical apprenticeship. Why not also teach *about* it? Why not admit phronesis, the practical epistemology of clinical medicine, as a legitimate field for investigation by physicians and medical students? The answer in part is that the current way of doing things works. Implicit or declared, the belief that medicine is a science remains useful as an ideal for physicians and patients alike—especially since, given the ethics of practice, it is seldom put unwaveringly into action. Instead, it endures unexamined and untested as an object of faith. Meanwhile, despite frequently disheartened students, dehumanized residents, burned-out physicians, dissatisfied patients, and stories about casual cruelty and real neglect, for most of us, most of the time, medicine works its miracles. Most days, for most of us, it ain't too broke.

And then there are the pedagogical reasons, strong arguments for not including medicine's practical epistemology in medical education and for describing it instead as a science. Even those physician-educators who know well that clinical practice is characterized by uncertainty, urgency, and imprecision may believe that only medicine's aspirations to be a science can promote and enforce sound rational procedures. Those who see clinical reasoning as inaccessibly unconscious can find the science claim a necessary counterweight to what cannot be described. And, as I have argued, experienced physicians may view the idealization of science as the best defense against emotion and subjectivity in medicine's intimate circumstances. All these arguments value clinical balance and the safety of patients, but they fail to appreciate the authority inherent in clinical medicine itself, an authority that is based in the acts of attention and care—including the very performance of certainty—in response to another human being's need.

A more worrisome reason for ignoring medicine's practical rationality is the possibility that self-knowledge is incapacitating. This is the "centipede problem," the belief that medicine cannot change and that it attempts to do so at its peril. The fear is that physicians, especially beginning ones, are like the centipede that was asked to explain how it walks. If they had to think about how they think, they might, like the centipede, be unable to take another step. Physicians must act—or decide not to act. If the status of clinical knowledge and its pervasive uncertainty were well described and understood, then thinking about thinking might make thought—or worse, effective action—impossible.

I have come to doubt this. Intellectual knowledge, including a thorough grasp of clinical thinking, is always trumped by the ethics of practice. This is true even for someone like the surgeon-writer, who thinks and writes about medicine's uncertainty. The reassurance he offered me after my daughter's illness came from his role as healer, and this is a role far more important, more integral to the person he is, than his interest in the status of his clinical knowledge. Thinking about our conversation that day has persuaded me that medicine's self-understanding can and ought to change. It can change because physicians are intelligent and fully capable of a reflective understanding of their work. It ought to change because, despite the hope and confidence conferred by their profession's identification with a simplistic conception of science, the costs of that identification are too great. The claim that medicine is a positivist science entails undesirable side effects for us all: for physicians, for society as a whole, and, above all, for patients and their families. Besides, medicine can change without risking physicians' capacity to act. Far from being like the fabled centipede, they are in no danger of sacrificing their clinical method—their deeply ingrained clinical habits—to mere theoretical knowledge, no matter how interesting or persuasive.

For physicians, the ethos of medical practice and the exercise of physicianly authority in patient care are far more habitual and compelling than any understanding of the status of their knowledge. Physicians, if asked, often acknowledge that clinical knowing is contingent and open to change. Only the customary irrelevance of thinking about it prevents their recognition of a gap between the profession's claim to be a science and the knowledge conditions of their actual practice. For those who recognize that gap, irony is the chief refuge.[23] For other clinicians, there is the "learned naïveté" that Pierre Bourdieu describes as characteristic of practices,[24] and this epistemological blind spot exists for the ironists, too, whenever they put on their white coats. As a consequence, there is no danger to patients or to physicians themselves from understanding how they think. Because medicine is not a science but a practice, its pedagogy is directed toward that practice rather than toward science—or philosophy, psychology, or cognitive theory. Like the human biology medical students spend so long learning, these other fields of knowledge provide reference points for the prepared mind but are not under immediate consideration. Students absorb instead the clinical habits and judgment necessary to patient care. If the medical profession asked its practitioners to think about how they think, and to examine the claim to be a science and the role of that assumption in medical education, clinical practice would not change. A profession-wide attention to clinical thinking would not challenge the acculturated blindness inherent in practice—just as clinical decision-making and evidence-based medicine have not done so. Theories about thinking and methods of knowing do not conflict with the ethics of medicine as a practice. They cannot. The ethics of patient care prevails.

The Ethics of Practice

Although medicine's ethics of practice outweighs whatever philosophical understanding clinicians have about their knowing, that ethics is often undervalued in the discourse of medicine. Despite its force—perhaps because that force is inalienable from practice—it is often ignored. Instead medicine's inherent values, exercised in the care of patients and inculcated throughout clinical education, are overlooked in favor of appeals to science as a warrant for clinical habits and attitudes and even for clinical decisions. But the values of science cannot substitute for medicine's own ethics of practice, nor are they the only way of achieving or reinforcing the behavioral goals of clinical education.

Medicine's ethics of practice calls first of all for the exercise of clinical judgment in response to a patient's need. It demands that physicians be thorough and careful observers. This is not because they are scientists, but because they are physicians caring for human beings who are ill. The ethics of practice also calls for an examination of the currency and reliability of one's knowledge—not because this is the duty of a scientist but because it is the obligation of all thinkers: historians, economists, and anthropologists, as well as physicians. Likewise, the ethics of practice values egalitarian openness, a characteristic so strong that institutions employing physicians put economic triage and financial gatekeepers between them and needy patients. Openness to all comers does not need scientific objectivity to justify it; it is part of medicine's identity as a profession. The ethics of practice also encourages a rigorous rationality and a commitment to continued learning, including an investigation of the reliability of current knowledge, not because medicine is a science but because its goal is good patient care. The ethics of practice also offers benefits that the ideal of science lacks. It provides comfort and protection for those caring for patients by acknowledging the human connection that is part of clinical work and not dooming them to think only of dissociated body parts. Above all, it encourages the acceptance of uncertainty and an appreciation of well-informed, well-exercised clinical judgment.

These values, inherent in the everyday care of patients, have shaped the methods used to teach clinical reasoning. There, in physicians' practical education, the virtues of honesty, attention, thoroughness, best effort, and skepticism are honed and rewarded. These are not virtues exclusive to science but general intellectual ones. They belonged to medicine long before there was much in the way of biological science, and, ideally, they are continually tempered and refined in beginning clinical students and experienced physicians alike. Throughout education and practice, cases are undertaken and reviewed. Those narrative representations of clinical judgment essential to acts of care are a powerful embodiment of clinical medicine's practical values.

Medicine's ethics of practice includes not only the values of attentive care but also a commitment to the continued refinement of clinical judgment. This, too, is not science but a pragmatism motivated by the duty to do one's best for the patient. Although scientific discoveries will continue to provide more (and more reliable) information, clinical knowing will remain unfinished and uncertain in the daily work of clinicians. However sophisticated their biomedical information, they will still have to figure out what is going on with every patient, one by one. This interpretive task requires a flexible cast of mind, a steady attention to the methods of practice, the habit of questioning, and a willingness to learn from others: observing, refining ideas, comparing notes. Such habits of mind are part of the ethics of practice, essential to becoming a physician and maintaining one's abilities over a lifetime. They may make clinical work feel like science even though this inferential clinical method is shared with all investigators—not excluding historians, psychologists, and musicologists—and resembles that of naturalists more than that of laboratory scientists. Increased scientific knowledge will not change either these procedures of clinical thinking or the values they represent. Evidence-based medicine, itself the product of clinical commitment and medicine's rational process, has challenged physicians to improve their clinical judgment with the use of more sophisticated statistical studies, but it has not displaced clinical medicine's fundamental rational, interpretive method. There is no need to label such devotion to knowledge "science," and, unlike its predecessors, evidence-based medicine has wisely avoided claiming it. It claims instead what is far more compelling: a curiosity about the universe of available information and a commitment to improve the individual clinician's practice.

In medicine, the ethics of practice is so strong that for physicians to understand how they think and work is unlikely to alter, much less impair, their clinical habits. Patient care comes first. For the clinician, theories of knowledge, like the understanding of scientific cause and even "facts" themselves, must serve a clinical purpose or they are not important, probably not even on the mental horizon. However important they may be at other times— "Uncertainty is my soap box!"—theories of knowing are set aside while the physician addresses the needs of the patient.

This is surely how an experienced clinician who had given a great deal of thought to the practice of medicine and was convinced of its inalienable uncertainty nevertheless could assure me that my daughter would not die of her disease. And my acceptance? A year later, reading Paul Auster's *Mr. Vertigo*, I came upon something like it. The novel is about a frontier magician, Master Yehudi, who is teaching a boy he plucked off the streets to fly. Step by step, trick by trick, the boy has launched himself into the air and become Mr. Vertigo. But when vigilantes murder the Native American woman who has been the boy's surrogate mother and the black child who has become his brother, the boy loses both the ability to fly and the desire to go on living. His teacher intervenes with the simplest, best trick of all. The dead pair come to him in dreams, Master Yehudi tells the boy; they are angels, now, singing and happy. The hero at first is deeply skeptical. But, whether through his need or his teacher's masterly performance or some combination of the two, the vision ultimately works:

> If the master lied, [the boy, now grown, tells us] then he did it for a reason. And if he didn't lie, then the story stands as told, and there's no cause to defend him. One way or the other, he saved me. One way or the other, he rescued my soul from the jaws of the beast.[25]

A year after my child's diagnosis, five months after her treatment ended, I didn't care about scientific fact or epidemiological probability. I heard a surgeon long in practice tell me my daughter would not die of breast cancer, and all the studies and statistics, the questions and data that I'd used for months to dismiss attempts to placate me died in my mouth. I leaned back in the passenger seat. It wasn't politeness or (except maybe for a split second) deference to someone who was giving me a ride to meet her. Instead, I was silenced by his assumption of a clinician's responsibility. It was not certainty he offered but his best judgment and the grounds on which he based it. It felt as solid as certainty and somehow more valuable because certainty, I knew, was not to be found. The situated particularity of his clinical judgment and, especially, his openness about its limits was oddly enough what made him trustworthy. Ironist that he no doubt was, he was not asking me to believe the facts, but him. Besides, her treatment was over; it was time.

In the next moment, I began to believe him. Something hard and despairing in me settled, quieted, then let go. "Thanks," I said provisionally, hearing it from a long way off—maybe just a little bit performatively. Then, unexpectedly, I saw that soon I would mean it with my whole heart.

NOTES

~~

Introduction

1. Renée Fox, "Training for Uncertainty," in *The Student-Physician*, ed. Robert Merton, George G. Reader, and Patricia L. Kendall (Cambridge, Mass.: Harvard University Press, 1957), pp. 207–41. Sherwin B. Nuland calls uncertainty "the muse that inspires the fascination of medical practice," in "The Uncertain Art: Proœmium," *American Scholar* 67 (spring 1998), 140.

2. Such rituals are nothing new: overdone, they have always provided the comedy in antimedical satire. Charles Bosk describes contemporary versions in "Occupational Rituals in Patient Management," *New England Journal of Medicine* 303 (1980), 71–76; and Jay Katz argues that physicians receive "training for [a façade of] certainty" in *The Silent World of Doctor and Patient* (New York: Free Press, 1984), p. 184.

3. Eric Cassell, *The Nature of Suffering and the Goals of Medicine* (New York: Oxford University Press, 1991), p. 76; Frederick W. Hafferty and Ronald Franks, "The Hidden Curriculum, Ethics Teaching and the Structure of Medical Education," *Academic Medicine* 69 (1994), 861–71.

4. Aristotle, *Nicomachean Ethics*, trans. Terence Irwin (Indianapolis: Hackett, 1985), 6.5–6. Irwin translates *phronesis* as "intelligence" and distinguishes it from wisdom and scientific knowledge (*sophia* and *episteme*).

5. Julian E. Orr, *Talking about Machines: An Ethnography of a Modern Job* (Ithaca: Cornell University Press, 1996).

6. *Phronesis* can be translated as "prudence," but the long history of that word's tight-lipped (and tight-fisted) use leads me to avoid it. By contrast, Edmund D. Pellegrino and David C. Thomasma, who call it "a sickly concept," admire the word's traditional use in translations of Aquinas and work to rehabilitate it; see *The Virtues in Medical Practice* (New York: Oxford University Press, 1993), p. 84.

7. Kirsti Malterud observes: "the traditional [bio]medical epistemology fails to represent medical knowledge adequately. The human interaction and interpretation which constitute a considerable element of clinical practice cannot be investigated from this epistemic position"; see "The Legitimacy of Clinical Knowledge: Towards a Medical Epistemology Embracing the Art of Medicine," *Theoretical Medicine* 16 (1995), 183.

8. In the 1980s, a spate of autobiographies about medical education described the punishing treatment of students and residents. See Perri Klass, *A Not Entirely Benign Procedure: Four Years as a Medical Student* (New York: Plume, 1994 [1987]);

Charles LeBaron, *Gentle Vengeance: An Account of the First Year at Harvard Medical School* (New York: Penguin, 1982); Melvin Konner, *Becoming a Doctor: A Journey of Initiation in Medical School* (New York: Viking, 1987); and, not least, the earlier satirical underground classic, Samuel Shem, *The House of God* (New York: Richard Marek, 1978), and Lawrence Schneiderman's comic *Sea Nymphs by the Hour* (Indianapolis: Bobbs Merrill, 1972). That they are not read avidly today and have few successors may be evidence of the success of curricular reforms.

9. Aristotle, *Metaphysics,* bk. 6.

10. Henry K. Silver, "Medical Students and Medical School," *Journal of the American Medical Association* 247 (1982), 309–10.

11. The Association of American Medical Colleges, *Physicians for the Twenty-First Century: The GPEP Report* (Washington, D.C. The Association of American Medical Colleges, 1984), inaugurated two decades of education reform. In 2001, the Accreditation Council on Graduate Medical Education (ACGME) decreed that for residents 80 hours a week on duty in a hospital is sufficient.

12. Kathryn Montgomery Hunter, *Doctors' Stories: The Narrative Structure of Knowledge in Medicine* (Princeton: Princeton University Press, 1991).

Chapter 1

Thanks to Catherine Belling, who invited me to present a version of this chapter in a session called "Authoring and Suffering: Agents and Patients, Ethics and Aesthetics in Medical Memoirs" at the annual meeting of the American Society for Bioethics and Humanities, Nashville, Tennessee, October 25, 2001, and to the audience who asked thoughtful questions about its implications for an epistemology of medicine.

1. Lynn Payer, *Medicine and Culture: Varieties of Treatment in the United States, England, West Germany, and France* (New York: Penguin Books, 1988), pp. 35–37, 27–28. See also Barron H. Lerner, *Breast Cancer Wars: Fear, Hope, and The Pursuit of a Cure in Twentieth-Century America* (New York: Oxford University Press, 2001).

2. In her dissertation, Gwynne Gertz explores the earlier 50-year lag in medical, particularly surgical, thinking between evidence supporting the modified radical mastectomy and the abandonment of the Halsted radical procedure; she finds similar patterns of resistance in the contemporary shift to the more recent lumpectomy and radiation. See " 'Whose Breast Is It Anyway?' A Change in Breast Cancer Discourse and Treatment," Ph.D. diss., University of Illinois, Chicago, 2003.

3. Daniel Kahneman and Amos Tversky, "The Framing of Decisions and the Psychology of Choice," *Science* 211 (1981), 453–58. See also their earlier "Judgment under Uncertainty," *Science* 185 (1974), 1124–31.

4. Stephen M. Cohen, " 'Kill the "probably," I said to myself. My sons need a father,' " *Johns Hopkins* (December 1980), 29–32.

5. Lewis Thomas, *The Youngest Science: Notes of a Medicine-Watcher* (New York: Viking, 1983). In fact, there are other, chronologically newer sciences—genetics and computer science, to name two—and were when Thomas wrote.

6. Aristotle, *Nicomachean Ethics*, trans. Terence Irwin, 2.2, 1104a7.

7. The legal analogues are legislation and case law.

8. George Engel, "A Need for a New Biomedical Model: A Challenge for Biomedicine," *Science* 196 (1977), 129–36.

9. Bernard Fisher, Stewart Anderson, John Bryant, Richard G. Margolese, Melvin Deutsch, Edwin R. Fisher, Jong-Hyeon Jeong, and Norman Wolmark, "Twenty-Year Follow-up of a Randomized Trial comparing Total Mastectomy, Lumpectomy, and Lumpectomy plus Irradiation for the Treatment of Invasive Breast Cancer," *New England Journal of Medicine* 347 (2002), 1233–41; and see the accompanying editorial by Monica Morrow, "Rational Local Treatment for Breast Cancer," 1270–71.

10. The occurrence is only 1 in 100,000, but breast cancer in men amounts to almost 1% of the breast cancer cases in the United States. Robert N. Riter describes the patient's experience in "I Have Breast Cancer," *Newsweek*, July 14, 1997, 14.

11. Lewis Thomas, *Lives of the Cell: Notes of a Biology Watcher* (New York: Viking Press, 1974). Thomas's description was in support of his plea for the value of basic biomedical research; since then, the HIV pandemic and the failure after 25 years to develop a vaccine has called those funding strategies into question; see Jon Cohen, *Shots in the Dark: The Wayward Search for an AIDS Vaccine* (New York: Norton, 2001).

12. Susan M. Love, Karen Lindsey, and Marcia Williams, *Dr. Susan Love's Breast Book*, 3rd rev. ed. (New York: HarperCollins, 2000).

13. Larry Dossey, *Healing Words: The Power of Prayer and the Practice of Medicine* (San Francisco: HarperCollins, 1994).

14. Rose Kushner, *Why Me? What Every Woman Should Know about Breast Cancer to Save Her Life* (New York: New American Library, 1977). See Barbara F. Sharf, "Out of the Closet and into the Legislature: The Impact of Communicating Breast Cancer Narratives on Health Policy," *Health Affairs* 20 (2001), 213–18.

15. Lester Grinspoon and James B. Bakalar, *Marihuana, the Forbidden Medicine* (New Haven: Yale University Press, 1993). Gould is quoted in their chapter on cancer treatment, p. 39.

16. David Spiegel and Catherine Classen, *Group Therapy for Cancer Patients: A Research Based Handbook of Psychosocial Care* (New York: Basic Books, 2000). Spiegel's work came to national attention in Bill Moyers's PBS television series *Healing and the Mind* (1993).

17. Audré Lorde, *The Cancer Journals* (Argyle, N.Y.: Spinsters Ink, 1980).

18. *New York Times Magazine*, August 15, 1993; see also http://www.matuschka.net/matuschka.html (accessed January 16, 2005).

Chapter 2

Parts of this chapter appeared in "Narrative, Literature, and the Clinical Exercise of Practical Reason," *Journal of Medicine and Philosophy* 21 (1996), 303–20, and in "Phronesis and the Misdescription of Medicine: Against *the* Medical School Commencement Speech," in *Bioethics: Ancient Themes in Contemporary Issues*, ed. Mark Kuczewski and Ronald Polansky (Cambridge, Mass.: MIT Press, 2000) pp. 57–66. I'm grateful to

Mark Waymack, who invited me to give the keynote address at the 1995 spring meeting of the Society for Health and Human Values, where I first tried out these ideas; to Mark Kuczewski, who included me in a panel presentation on bioethics and classical philosophy at the American Philosophical Society meeting in Chicago, and to Anne Hunsaker Hawkins, who coedited that interestingly contentious 1996 issue of *Journal of Medicine and Philosophy*.

1. Henry E. Sigerest, *On the History of Medicine*, ed. Felix Marti-Ibanez (New York: MD, 1960).

2. Marsden Scott Blois criticizes this phenomenon and includes a list of notable examples in his fine essay "Medicine and the Nature of Vertical Reasoning," *New England Journal of Medicine* 318 (1988), 847–51.

3. Kirsti Malterud challenges this neglect in "The Legitimacy of Clinical Knowledge: Towards a Medical Epistemology Embracing the Art of Medicine," *Theoretical Medicine* 16 (1995), 183–98. She defines the art of medicine as "the successful interrelationship between the biomedical and the humanistic perspectives in clinical practice," which includes the researchable domains of "human interaction in clinical contexts, clinical judgment and reasoning, and clinical philosophy" (189).

4. Donald Schön, *Educating the Reflective Practitioner: Toward a New Design for Teaching and Learning in the Professions* (San Francisco: Jossey-Bass, 1987), p. 13. Writing about practical knowledge generally, Schön uses "art" for the capacity for problem-framing, implementation, and improvisation: what he terms "knowing-in-action."

5. Kenneth Schaffner, *Discovery and Explanation in Biology and Medicine* (Chicago: University of Chicago Press, 1994).

6. A. C. Dornhurst asserts that medicine is "science-using" rather than a science in "Information Overload: Why Medical Education Needs a Shake-up," *Lancet* 2 (1981), 513–14.

7. Aristotle, *Metaphysics*, bk. 6. See also Kathryn Montgomery Hunter, "A Science of Individuals: Medicine and Casuistry," *Journal of Medicine and Philosophy* 14 (1989), 193–212, a version of which appears as chapter 2 of *Doctors' Stories* (Princeton: Princeton University Press, 1991).

8. Caroline A. Jones and Peter Galison, introduction to *Picturing Science, Producing Art* (New York: Routledge: 1998), p. 2. See also D. Graham Burnett, "A View from the Bridge: The Two Cultures Debate, Its Legacy, and the History of Science," *Daedalus* 128 (spring 1999), 193–218.

9. Edmund D. Pellegrino and David C. Thomasma describe phronesis as "medicine's indispensable virtue," in *The Virtues in Medical Practice* (New York: Oxford University Press, 1993), pp. 84–91. They maintain a distinction between practical reason and clinical judgment—"clinical judgment is essentially the exercise of prudence" (86)—while my argument follows ordinary usage in taking "judgment" to mean both a capacity or virtue and its exercise. Earlier they had identified "prudent and judicious action" as the end of clinical judgment; see *A Philosophical Basis of Medical Practice : Toward a Philosophy and Ethic of the Healing Professions* (New York: Oxford University Press, 1981), p. 121, and they continue to make use of the word's ambiguity when they speak of phronesis as "the virtue of practical judgment" (*Virtues*, p. 184).

10. Aristotle, *Nicomachean Ethics*, 2.2, 1104a7.

11. Case-based reasoning is the most promising area of research; see Roger C. Schank and Robert P. Abelson, *Scripts, Plans, Goals and Understanding: An Inquiry into Human Knowledge* (Hillsdale, N.J.: Erlbaum, 1981); Roger C. Schank, *Tell Me a Story: A New Look at Real and Artificial Memory* (New York: Scribners, 1990); Janet Kolodner, *Case-Based Reasoning* (Palo Alto, Calif.: Morgan Kaufmann, 1993); and Kristian Hammond, *Case-Based Planning: Viewing Planning as a Memory Task* (Boston: Academic Press, 1989).

12. John Lantos considers this, among other reasons, in *Do We Still Need Doctors?* (New York: Routledge, 1997).

13. Patricia Benner, *From Novice to Expert: Excellence and Power in Clinical Nursing Practice* (Reading, Mass.: Addison-Wesley, 1984).

14. Hubert L. Dreyfus and Stuart E. Dreyfus, "From Socrates to Expert Systems: The Limits of Calculative Rationality," in *Interpretive Social Sciences: A Second Look*, ed. Paul Rabinow and William M. Sullivan (Berkeley: University of California Press, 1987), pp. 327–50. They quote Edward Feigenbaum and Pamela McCorduck, *The Fifth Generation: Artificial Intelligence and Japan's Computer Challenge* (Reading, Mass.: Addison-Wesley, 1983), p. 82.

15. David L. Sackett, Sharon E. Straus, W. Scott Richardson, William Rosenberg, and R. Brian Haynes, *Evidence Based Medicine*, 2nd ed. (New York: Churchill Livingstone, 2000). See also Alvan Feinstein, *Clinimetrics* (New Haven: Yale University Press, 1987).

16. This point has been made by Michael Alan Schwartz and Osborne Wiggins with regard to the biomedical model that George Engel famously found wanting; "Science, Humanism, and the Nature of Medical Practice: A Phenomenological View," *Perspectives in Biology and Medicine* 28 (1985), 334.

17. Malterud, "Legitimacy," p. 183.

18. Eric Cassell, *The Nature of Suffering and the Goals of Medicine* (New York: Oxford University Press, 1991), p. xi. His 1997 *Doctoring: The Nature of Primary Care Medicine* (New York: Oxford University Press), an experience-based epistemology of medicine, describes the inadequacy of science—its "superficiality"—as a model and a source for clinical knowing.

19. Edmund D. Pellegrino and David C. Thomasma, *A Philosophical Basis of Medical Practice*, pp. 125–43.

20. The Cochane Collaboration is available online at: www.cochrane.org (accessed September 15, 2004).

21. Linda T. Kohn, Janet M. Corrigan, and Molla S. Donaldson, eds., *To Err Is Human: Building a Safer Health System* (Washington, D.C.: Committee on Quality of Health Care in America, Institute of Medicine, 2000).

22. Hans-Georg Gadamer, *The Enigma of Health: The Art of Healing in a Scientific Age*, trans. Jason Gaiger and Nicholas Walker (Stanford: Stanford University Press, 1996), p. 4.

23. Harold Bursztajn, Richard I. Feinbloom, Robert M. Hamm, and Archie Brodsky describe how it might be done in *Medical Choices, Medical Chances*, 2nd ed. (New York: Routledge, 1990).

24. Charles Bosk, *Forgive and Remember: Managing Medical Failure* (Chicago: University of Chicago Press, 1979). See also Pellegrino and Thomasma, *Philosophical Basis of Medical Practice.*

Chapter 3

Early versions of the argument of this chapter were presented as "Medicine Is Not a Science: Rationality in an Uncertain Practice," the 1998 Osler Lecture at McGill University, and as "Medicine and the Masque of Science," the 1998 Harriet Sheridan Literature and Medicine Lecture at Brown University. I'm grateful to Abraham Fuks, dean of the Medical School at McGill, and to Lynn Epstein, associate dean of medical education at Brown, for their invitations. Parts of this chapter have appeared in "Narrative, Literature, and the Clinical Exercise of Practical Reason," *Journal of Medicine and Philosophy* 21 (1996), 303–20, and in "Phronesis and the Misdescription of Medicine: Against *the* Medical School Commencement Speech," *Bioethics: Ancient Themes in Contemporary Issues*, ed. Mark Kuczewski and Ronald Polansky (Cambridge, Mass.: MIT Press, 2000), pp. 57–66.

1. The phenomenologist Richard Zaner once lamented that the principles of medical ethics were developed without a thorough description of clinical practice: "Only a handful of serious efforts," he observed, "have been made to understand the complicated discipline of medicine"; see Richard M. Zaner, "Experience and Moral Life: A Phenomenological Approach to Bioethics," in Edward R. DuBose, R. P. Hamel, Lawrence J. O'Connell, eds. *A Matter of Principles? Ferment in U.S. Bioethics* (Valley Forge, Pa.: Trinity Press International, 1994), pp. 211–39.

2. David L. Sackett, Sharon E. Straus, W. Scott Richardson, William Rosenberg, R. Brian Haynes, *Evidence Based Medicine*, 2nd ed. (New York: Churchill Livingstone, 2000).

3. Excellent work has been done on the psychology of clinical reasoning; see Alvan Feinstein, *Clinical Judgment* (Baltimore: Williams and Wilkins, 1967); Arthur S. Elstein, Lee S. Shulman, Sarah A. Sprafka, *Medical Problem Solving: An Analysis of Clinical Reasoning* (Cambridge, Mass.: Harvard University Press, 1978); Patricia Benner, *From Novice to Expert: Excellence and Power in Clinical Nursing Practice* (Reading, Mass.: Addison-Wesley, 1984); Georges Bordage and Madeleine Lemieux, "Semantic Structures and Diagnostic Thinking of Experts and Novices," *Academic Medicine* 66 (1990), S70-S72; Jerome P. Kassirer and Richard I. Kopelman, *Learning Clinical Reasoning* (Baltimore: Williams and Wilkins, 1991); Geoffrey R. Norman, "The Non-Analytical Basis of Clinical Reasoning," presented to the Case-Based Reasoning Group in the Department of Computer Science, University of Chicago, December 14, 1994.

4. Aristotle, *Nicomachean Ethics*, trans. Terence Irwin (Indianapolis: Hackett, 1985), 2.2, 1104a.

5. "[T]he latter kind of thinking is . . . in the main derived from our actual experience of the order of things . . . in the real outward world"; see William James,

"Brute and Human Intellect [1878]," in *Writings 1878–1899* (New York: Viking, 1992), p. 911. Jerome Bruner uses James's distinction as the epigraph for *Actual Minds, Possible Worlds* (Cambridge, Mass.: Harvard University Press, 1986).

6. Although they have not altered medicine's use of an ideal drawn from older concepts, particularly of the physical sciences, historians and philosophers of science have demonstrated that scientists reason contextually and interpretively; see Bruno Latour and Steve Woolgar, *Laboratory Life: The Construction of Scientific Facts* (Beverly Hills, Calif.: Sage, 1979; reprint, Princeton University Press, 1986); Mary Hesse, "Texts without Types, Lumps without Laws," *New Literary History* 17 (1985), 31–48; Helen E. Longino, *Science as Social Knowledge: Values and Objectivity in Scientific Inquiry* (Princeton: Princeton University Press, 1990).

7. John Dewey, *Human Nature and Conduct: An Introduction to Social Psychology* (1922), in *The Middle Works, 1899–1924*, vol. 14 (Carbondale: Southern Illinois State University Press, 1988); see also *The Quest for Certainty: A Study of the Relation of Knowledge and Action* (1929), in *The Later Works, 1925–53*, vol. 1 (Carbondale: Southern Illinois State University Press, 1981).

8. Hilary Putnam, "The Craving for Objectivity," *New Literary History* 15 (1984), 229–39.

9. Clifford Geertz, *Local Knowledge: Further Essays in Interpretative Anthropology* (New York: Basic Books, 1983); Stanley Jeyaraja Tambiah, *Magic, Science, Religion, and the Scope of Rationality* (New York: Cambridge University Press, 1990).

10. Hayden White, "The Value of Narrativity in the Representation of Reality," *Critical Inquiry* 7 (1980), 5–27, reprinted in *On Narrative*, ed. W.J.T. Mitchell (Chicago: University of Chicago Press, 1980), pp. 1–23; Dominick La Capra, *History, Politics, and the Novel* (Ithaca: Cornell University Press, 1987).

11. Jerome Bruner, *Actual Minds, Possible Worlds* (Cambridge, Mass.: Harvard University Press, 1986). See also Katherine Nelson, ed., *Narratives from the Crib* (Cambridge, Mass.: Harvard University Press, 1989). In *Consciousness Explained* (Boston: Little, Brown, 1991), philosopher of mind Daniel Dennett describes the source of the self in brain-created narratives.

12. Charles Taylor, *Sources of the Self: The Making of Modern Identity* (Cambridge, Mass.: Harvard University Press, 1989), pp. 7, 74–75.

13. In his epistemology of practice, Donald A. Schön describes this as the dilemma of rigor and relevance; see *Educating the Reflective Practitioner: Toward a New Design for Teaching and Learning in the Professions* (San Francisco: Jossey-Bass, 1987), p. xi.

14. On the alienation of bioethics from clinical judgment see David J. Rothman, *Strangers at the Bedside: A History of How Law and Bioethics Transformed Medical Decision Making* (New York: Basic Books, 1991). Robert Zussman, *Intensive Care: Medical Ethics and the Medical Profession* (Chicago: University of Chicago Press, 1992), documents the attempts of critical care physicians to preserve ethical decisions as an aspect of professional expertise.

15. Ronald J. Allen, my law school colleague, pointed this out to me. Arguing for narrative plausibility between "equally well-specified cases" as the standard for evidence in "The Nature of Juridical Proof," *Cardozo Law Review* 13 (1991), 373–422, he describes the epistemological clash in legal fact-finding between a conceptually

driven ("episode") method of knowing and a data-driven ("elements") one. As he compares law with other fields of knowledge, his survey of handbooks of clinical diagnosis leads him to liken medicine to data-driven analytical chemistry rather than to conceptually driven historiography. It is more probable that, like the instructions judges give to juries, diagnostic textbooks impose a data-driven method on what is inescapably a conceptual or narrative way of knowing. Whether the "scientism" of diagnostic textbooks and judges' instructions to juries is wholly a matter of misunderstanding or a necessary counterbalance deserves study.

16. C. S. Peirce, "Abduction and Induction," in *Philosophical Writings of Peirce*, ed. Justus Buchler (New York: Dover, 1955). See also Umberto Eco and Thomas A. Sebeok, eds., *The Sign of The Three: Dupin, Holmes, Peirce* (Bloomington: Indiana University Press, 1983).

17. I use "narrative" interchangeably with "story" to designate a historical or fictional account of occurrences, whether written, spoken, or performed. The terms, however, have different connotations: "narrative," used for both nonfiction and fiction, sometimes suggests a contrast with visual or numerical data; the homelier word "story" often denotes spoken or fictional accounts; it always implies the existence of a storyteller. This definition, with much of the description in the next two paragraphs, appears in "Narrative," *Encyclopedia of Bioethics*, 2nd ed., ed. Warren T. Reich (New York: Macmillan, 1995), pp. 1789–94.

18. Alasdair MacIntyre, *After Virtue: A Study in Moral Theory* (South Bend, Ind.: Notre Dame University Press, 1981).

19. Anne Hunsaker Hawkins, *Reconstructing Illness: Studies in Pathography*, 2nd ed. (West Lafayette, Ind.: Purdue University Press, 1999; Arthur W. Frank, "Reclaiming an Orphan Genre: The First-Person Narrative of Illness," *Literature and Medicine* 13 (1994) 1–21.

20. Patricia Meyer Spacks, *Gossip* (New York: Knopf, 1985); See also Michelle Z. Rosaldo, "Toward an Anthropology of Self and Feeling," in *Culture Theory*, ed. Richard A. Shweder and Robert E. LeVine (Cambridge: Cambridge University Press, 1984), pp. 137–57.

21. Cases only seem objective, a quality they simultaneously claim and strive for. The medical knower (sometimes the teller, sometimes a whole team of clinicians) is nevertheless the central consciousness; we learn facts about the patient in a standardized way, just as that knower was trained to become aware of and record them.

22. In opposition to structuralist and semiotic theorists, Paul Ricoeur argues that time is essential to narrative: *Time and Narrative*, 3 vols., trans. Kathleen McLaughlin Blamey and David Pellauer (Chicago: University of Chicago Press, 1984–88).

23. Martha C. Nussbaum, *The Fragility of Goodness: Luck and Ethics in Greek Tragedy and Philosophy* (New York: Cambridge University Press, 1986); Bernard Williams, *Moral Luck: Philosophical Papers, 1973–1980* (New York: Cambridge University Press, 1981).

24. Wayne C. Booth, *The Company We Keep: An Ethics of Fiction* (Berkeley: University of California Press, 1988).

25. Stanley Hauerwas and David Burrell, "From System to Story: An Alternative Pattern for Rationality in Ethics" [1977], in *Why Narrative? Readings in Narrative The-*

ology, ed. L. Gregory Jones and Stanley Hauerwas (Grand Rapids, Mich.: Eerdmans, 1989), pp. 158–90.

26. Aristotle, *Nicomachean Ethics*, trans. Terence Irwin (Indianapolis: Hackett, 1985), 6.8.

27. Stephen Toulmin, "Knowledge and Art in the Practice of Medicine: Clinical Judgment and Historical Reconstruction," in *Science, Technology, and the Art of Medicine*, ed. Corrina Delkeskamp-Hayes and Mary Ann Gardell Cutter (Dordrect: Kluwer, 1993), pp. 231–49.

28. See Cass R. Sunstein's defense of nonpropositional analogical reasoning in law, "On Analogical Reasoning," *Harvard Law Review* 106 (1993), 741–91. He quotes at length Mary Hesse's skeptical account of the way we think we reason:

> It has long been obvious that the human problem solver does not generally think deductively or by exhaustive search of logical space. Propositional logic relies upon enumeration of premises, univocal symbolization, and exclusively deductive connections, and these cannot be either a good simulation of human thought or an efficient use of computers. In real human thinking, the meanings of concepts are constantly modified and extended by parallels, models and metaphors, and the rational steps from premises to conclusion are generally non-demonstrative, being carried out by inductive, hypothetical and analogical reasoning.

See her "Family Resemblances and Analogy," in *Analogical Reasoning: Perspectives of Artificial Intelligence, Cognitive Science, and Philosophy*, ed. David H. Helman (Dordrecht: Kluwer, 1988), pp. 317–18.

29. Renée Fox, "Training for Uncertainty," in *The Student-Physician*, ed. Robert Merton, George G. Reader, and Patricia L. Kendall (Cambridge, Mass.: Harvard University Press, 1957), pp. 207–41.

30. Hans-Georg Gadamer, maintaining that practical wisdom is not (as Giambattisto Vico implied) a matter of probabilistic reasoning, cites Helmholtz's description of this mode of knowing as "a kind of tact" that is as judicious in its omissions as in its selection of experiential information; *Truth and Method*, 2nd ed. (New York: Crossroad, 1984), pp. 16–17.

Chapter 4

1. Causality, of course, is a far more complicated question, especially in physics, where laws are bidirectional and timeless, and in probability theory, which has no place for it. Cause nevertheless remains a useful empirical concept. Judea Pearl, "The Art and Science of Cause and Effect," describes a mathemathical model for experimental intervention, an "algebra of doing" that makes possible "a causal understanding of poverty and cancer and intolerance" and, it seems to me, a genuinely postmodern science of medicine. The lecture is reprinted as epilogue to his *Causality: Models, Reasoning, and Inference* (Cambridge: Cambridge University Press, 2000), pp. 331–58.

2. The other three causes Aristotle identified are material cause (the substance of a thing), formal cause (its shape or pattern), and final cause (its purpose or reason for being).

3. The Sherlock Holmes stories offer evidence for this historical continuity. Written between 1883 and 1927, they nevertheless exhibit the principal characteristics of clinical reasoning.

4. Eric Cassell, who first problematized the concept of cause in medicine in his optimistic "Changing Ideas of Causality in Medicine," *Social Research* 46 (1979), 728–43, bluntly declared a dozen years later, "Physicians do not treat causes; they use drugs and surgery to restore performance or relieve dysfunction in a manner specific to the problem"; *The Nature of Suffering and the Goals of Medicine* (New York: Oxford University Press, 1991), p. 92.

5. Arthur Conan Doyle gives Sherlock Holmes this capacity, and it is almost certainly the reason so many physicians are fans of the detective. See, for example, Holmes's rapid identification of the retired sergeant of marines in *A Study in Scarlet* or his rather typical complaint in "The Blue Carbuncle" that explanation makes such a feat seem ordinary, a commonsense perception available to all comers. The phrase "tacit knowledge" is from Michael Polanyi, *Personal Knowledge: Toward a Post-Critical Philosophy* [1958] (Chicago: University of Chicago Press, 1971), p. 264.

6. Julia E. Connelly and Alvin Mushlin, "The Reasons Patients Request 'Check-ups,' " *Journal of General Internal Medicine* 1 (1986), 163–65; the study finds that requests for a physical examination are most often motivated by substantial worry.

7. The term *normal discourse* is Richard Rorty's in *Philosophy and the Mirror of Nature* (Princeton: Princeton University Press, 1979). Rorty adapts this idea from Thomas Kuhn's description of "normal" and "abnormal science" in *The Structure of Scientific Revolutions*, 2nd ed. (Chicago: University of Chicago Press, 1970), p. 11. Compare the introduction of the "abnormal discourse" of AIDS or toxic shock syndrome in the early 1980s or chronic fatigue syndrome in the 1990s.

8. See chapter 10 for discussion of common sense.

9. Georg Henrik von Wright, *Explanation and Understanding* (Ithaca: Cornell University Press, 1971).

10. Raymond H. Curry inspired this observation, and I am indebted to him for the discussion that provoked it.

11. Jerome Groopman, *The Measure of Our Days: A Spiritual Exploration of Illness* (New York: Penguin Books, 1997), pp. 9.

12. Alvan R. Feinstein introduced these concepts to medicine in *Clinical Judgment* (Huntington, N.Y.: Krieger, 1967).

13. Bayes's theorem, which was derived from a posthumously published essay by the eighteenth-century English clergyman, Thomas Bayes, supplies a formula for revising probabilities as new data become available. Used by web search engines like Google, its theory of inference gives physicians a means of incorporating background knowledge in determining the usefulness and reliability of tests for particular patients. Despite the approximate certainty implied by its mathematical representation, Bayesian inference, like statistics more generally, informs clinical judgment but is never a substitute for it.

14. Michael Bérubé, *Life as We Know It: A Father, a Family, and an Exceptional Child* (New York: Pantheon Books, 1996).

15. John Ladd, "Philosophy and Medicine," in *Changing Values in Medicine*, ed. Eric J. Cassell and Mark Siegler (Frederick, Md.: University Publications, n.d.[1985]), p. 213.

16. It happens, of course, and, when it does, it generates stories—even in subspecialties where physicians see a narrowed range of patients in their area of expertise; see, for example, the dermatologist's story, p. 109.

17. Marsden S. Blois, *Information and Medicine: The Nature of Medical Descriptions* (Berkeley: University of California Press, 1984).

18. By all accounts, the connection of *helicobacter* with peptic ulcers is medical science of the lonely pioneering kind that is viewed with some suspicion by sociologists of knowledge. An Australian researcher ingested *helicobacter* to prove what his colleagues had been reluctant to credit; he got an ulcer. There were, of course, a lab and a network of researchers, a journal, newspapers, and, above all, physicians eager for a better answer to the puzzle of a hard-to-treat condition. See Barry Marshall, ed., *Helicobacter Pioneers* (Oxford: Blackwell Scientific, 2002).

Chapter 5

1. Kenneth Schaffner, *Discovery and Explanation in Biology and Medicine* (Chicago: University of Chicago, 1994). Stephen Toulmin compares "everyday . . . causation" and "medical causation" and finds that science has not changed the latter in "Causation and the Locus of Medical Intervention," in *Changing Values in Medicine*, ed. Eric J. Cassell and Mark Siegler (Frederick, Md: University Publications, n.d.[1985]), pp. 59–72. Marsden S. Blois illustrates the multilevel nature of medical reasoning in "Medicine and the Nature of Vertical Reasoning," *New England Journal of Medicine* 318 (1988), 847–51.

2. David Morris, *Illness and Culture in the Postmodern Age* (Berkeley: University of California Press, 2000).

3. See Ludwig von Bertalanffy, *General Systems Theory* (New York: Braziller, 1968); George L. Engel, "The Need for a New Biomedical Model: A Challenge for Biomedicine," *Science* 196 (1977), 129–36; and Blois, "Medicine and the Nature of Vertical Reasoning," 847–51.

4. Lewis White Beck, personal communication, 1983; Stephen Toulmin includes a version of this story in "Causation and the Locus of Medical Intervention," pp. 59–60.

5. Georg Henrik von Wright calls this quasi-teleological causality; see *Explanation and Understanding* (Ithaca: Cornell University Press, 1971). Contrast this with quasi-causal teleology, p. 63.

6. On the tension between physiological and ontological conceptions of illness and disease, see Eric Cassell, "Ideas in Conflict: The Rise and Fall of New Views of Disease," in *The Nature of Suffering and the Goals of Medicine* (New York: Oxford University Press, 1991), pp. 3–16, and Julia Epstein, *Altered Conditions: Disease, Medicine, and Storytelling* (New York: Routledge, 1994).

7. In people of northern European descent, the CCR5 mutation from one parent confers resistance; from both parents, it confers immunity. Thanks to Robert Hirschtick for this example.

8. Richard Rorty, *Philosophy and the Mirror of Nature* (Princeton: Princeton University Press, 1979), p. 11.

9. Robert A. Aronowitz, *Making Sense of Illness: Science, Society and Disease* (Cambridge: Cambridge University Press, 1998). I'm grateful to Andrew Cohen for this book.

10. Or consider the experience of teaching someone to drive a car. Expert knowledge, including clinical intuition, is discussed in chapters 7 and 9.

11. Carlo Ginzburg, "Clues: Roots of an Evidential Paradigm," in *Clues, Myths, and the Historical Method*, trans. John and Anne Tedeschi (Baltimore: Johns Hopkins University Press, 1986; the emphasis is Ginzburg's.

12. Not that there haven't been attempts to make history a science: chief among them are the midcentury French historians associated with *Annales* and the philosopher Carl G. Hempel in his essay "The Function of General Laws in History," *Journal of Philosophy* 39 (1942). The closest analogue to medicine may be "cliometricians," historians who base their interpretation on economic data; see, for example, Robert William Fogel and Stanley L. Engerman's groundbreaking and controversial *Time on the Cross: The Economics of Negro Slavery* (Boston: Little Brown, 1974).

13. Edmund D. Pellegrino and David C. Thomasma, *A Philosophical Basis of Medical Practice: Toward a Philosophy and Ethics of the Healing Professions* (New York: Oxford University Press, 1981), pp. 125–43.

14. National Commission for the Protection of Human Subjects of Biomedical and Behavioral Research, *The Belmont Report: Ethical Principles and Guidelines for the Protections of Human Subjects of Research* (Washington, D.C.: U.S. Government Printing Office, 1978).

15. Bruno Latour, *We Have Never Been Modern*, trans. Katherine Porter (Cambridge, Mass.: Harvard University Press, 1993), p. 6.

16. Kathryn Montgomery Hunter, "Eating the Curriculum: Metaphors for Medical Education," *Academic Medicine*, 72 (1997), 167–72. The Accreditation Council on Graduate Medical Education has taken steps to change residency education; see www.acgme.org/outcome/comp/compFull.asp (accessed May 5, 2004).

Chapter 6

An early version of this chapter was presented at the International Bioethics Retreat in Almagro, Spain, June 4, 2002. The rumination on solitaire was the subject of an earlier Medical Humanities and Bioethics Work-in-Progress Group meeting at Northwestern University.

1. In reality, of course, scientists are practical reasoners, too, since their thinking is far more complex and contextualized than the idealized picture of scientific work that inspires medicine; see notes on the history and philosophy of science, p. 215 n6.

2. Katherine Nelson, ed., *Narratives from the Crib* (Cambridge, Mass.: Harvard University Press, 1989).

3. Aristotle, *Metaphysics*, bk. 6.

4. John Wisdom tells this story in *Paradox and Certainty* (Oxford: Blackwell, 1965), p. 138. I'm grateful to Tod Chambers for finding the source.

5. David L. Sackett, Sharon E. Straus, W. Scott Richardson, William Rosenberg, and R. Brian Haynes, *Evidence Based Medicine*, 2nd ed. (New York: Churchill Livingstone, 2000).

6. See Mark R. Tonelli, "The Philosophical Limits of EBM," *Academic Medicine* 73 (1998), 1234–40, and Trisha Greenhalgh, "Narrative Based Medicine in an Evidence Based World," *British Medical Journal* 318 (1999), 323–25; reprinted in *Narrative Based Medicine*, ed. Trisha Greenhalgh and Brian Hurwitz (London: British Medical Journal Press, 1999), pp. 247–65. A third charge, that EBM is impractically time-consuming, depends on the clinician's facility with internet searches and the quality of the technology used. But see W. Scott Richardson and Steven D. Burdette, "Practice Corner: Taking Evidence in Hand," from *ACP Journal Club* 138 (2003), pp. A9–10, which describes the use of EBM on a morning's rounds including—along with questions, methods, and sources found—a record of the time spent on each search.

7. Hunches, anecdotally reported, deserve study. Atul Gawande tells of deciding against amputating a young woman's leg when missing the diagnosis of necrotizing fasciitis would have meant her death: "It is still not apparent to me what the clues were that I was registering when I first saw Eleanor's leg. Likewise, it is not obvious what the signs were that we could get by without an amputation." See "The Case of the Red Leg," in *Complications: A Surgeon's Notes on an Imperfect Science* (New York: Metropolitan, 2002), pp. 228–52. Trisha Greenhalgh tells of a general practitioner, Dr. Jenkins, who learns that a patient he knows well has called to say her daughter has diarrhea and is "behaving strangely." He leaves his office—this is England—and arrives in time to diagnose and treat the child's meningococcal meningitis, a dread disease he had only seen once in almost 100,000 patient visits. See "Narrative Based Medicine in an Evidence Based World."

8. John Ladd argues that this inseparability of discovery from justification is one of clinical medicine's principal differences from science; see "Philosophy and Medicine," in *Changing Values in Medicine*, ed. Eric J. Cassell and Mark Siegler ([Frederick, Md.: University Publications, n.d. [1985]). By contrast, Koch's postulates require biomedical scientists to confirm a diagnosis by transferring the disease to another subject.

9. This was illustrated in early 2003 when the rapid identification of the SARS coronavirus was regarded as complete only after, following Koch's postulates, serum from a patient was injected into primates and produced the same symptoms and the same viral profile.

10. Alvan Feinstein, "*Clinical Judgment* Revisited: The Distraction of Quantitative Models," *Annals of Internal Medicine* 120 (1994), 799–805.

11. See Thomas McLaughlin, *Street Smarts and Critical Theory: Listening to the Vernacular* (Madison: University of Wisconsin Press, 1996).

12. This term and the adjective "multiplicative" hereafter are Howard S. Becker's. I am indebted throughout this chapter to his *Tricks of the Trade* (Chicago: University

of Chicago Press, 1998), a guide to research in the social sciences and a masterpiece of pragmatic epistemology.

13. Conversely, if the patient's history does not include such causal clues, those possibilities are moved, with residual skepticism, to the bottom of the list ("patient denies alcohol and drug use"), and diagnostic tests for those less likely conditions, if they are done, will be far less reliable.

14. Robert A. Aronowitz, *Making Sense of Illness: Science, Society and Disease* (Cambridge: Cambridge University Press, 1998).

15. Harold Kushner made randomness somewhat more acceptable in *When Bad Things Happen to Good People* (New York: Schoecken Books, 1981).

16. None of her informants attributed their illness to "luck" while an overwhelming majority in the United States saw "stress" as the medico-moral term mediating between mind (or soul) and body; see Grace Gredys Harris, "Mechanism and Morality in Patients' Views of Illness and Injury," *Medical Anthropology Quarterly,* n.s. 3 (1989), 3–21. See also her *Casting Out Anger: Religion among the Taita of Kenya* (Cambridge: Cambridge University Press, 1978).

Chapter 7

Early versions of this chapter were presented to the Case-Based Reasoning Group in the Computer Science Department at the University of Chicago, an ethics seminar at Indiana University Medical School, the joint Duke–University of North Carolina medical ethics study group, and the spring 1996 meeting of the Society for Health and Human Values. My thanks to Jeffrey Berger, Kristian Hammond, John Woodcock, Nancy M. P. King, and Hilde Lindemann Nelson for their invitations. A version appeared as "Aphorisms, Maxims, and Old Saws: Narrative Rationality and the Negotiation of Clinical Choice," in *Stories and their Limits,* ed. Hilde Lindemann Nelson (New York: Routledge, 1997), pp. 215–31. The story of the 40-year-old man with endocarditis appeared in " 'Don't Think Zebras': Uncertainty, Interpretation, and the Place of Paradox in Clinical Education," *Theoretical Medicine* 5 (1996), 1–17, and was reprinted by Trisha Greenhalgh, with additional clinical examples of conflicting maxims, in her "Narrative Based Medicine in an Evidence Based World," *Narrative Based Medicine,* ed. Trisha Greenhalgh and Brian Hurwitz (London: BMJ Press, 1999), pp. 247–65.

1. Arthur Elstein and his colleagues established that diagnostic skill does not exist without the relevant clinical information; Arthur S. Elstein, Lee S. Shulman, Sarah A. Sprafka, *Medical Problem Solving: An Analysis of Clinical Reasoning* (Cambridge, Mass.: Harvard University Press, 1978).

2. National Comprehensive Cancer Network, "Locoregional Treatment of Clinical Stage I, IIA, or IIB Disease or T3,N1, M0," *Clinical Practice Guidelines in Oncology* [online] 1 (2005). Available online at: www.nccn.org (accessed April 10, 2005), p. 10.

3. Clifton K. Meador, *A Little Book of Doctors' Rules* (Philadelphia: Hanley and Belfus, 1992). Frank Davidoff writes about aphorisms in "A Technology for Remembering: Aphorisms and Maxims," in *Who Has Seen a Blood Sugar? Reflections on Medical Education* (Philadelphia: American College of Physicians, 1996). I am grateful to Ann Folwell Stanford for the first and to Raymond H. Curry for the second. Most, but not all, of the sayings in this chapter were gathered in departments of internal medical in several medical schools. There are trends in aphorisms, as with all colloquialisms, and they are influenced by time and powerful speakers.

4. This claim is often made in conversation and in print without citation—as if not only the claim but the percentages alleged were common knowledge. Lynn Payer attributes one such claim—of 75%—to Dr. Donald Young of the Mayo Clinic, in her *Medicine and Culture* (New York: Penguin), p. 141. An actual study that yielded 82% is reported by J. R. Hampton, M.J.G. Harrison, J.R.A. Mitchell, J. S. Prichard, and Carol Seymour, "Relative Contributions of History-Taking, Physical Examination, and Laboratory Investigation to Diagnosis and Management of Medical Outpatients," *British Medical Journal* 2 (1975), 486–89. I'm grateful to Bill Donnelly for this reference.

5. Marsden S. Blois, *Information and Medicine: The Nature of Medical Descriptions* (Berkeley: University of California Press, 1984), p. 165. And see Lawrence L. Weed, *Medical Records, Medical Education, & Patient Care: The Problem-Oriented Medical Record* (Cleveland: The Press of Case Western Reserve University, 1971).

6. As Leon Edel observed, "The biographer may be as imaginative as he pleases— the more imaginative the better—in the way in which he brings together his materials, but he must not imagine the materials"; quoted by James Atlas, "When Fact Is Treated as Fiction," *New York Times, News of the Week in Review,* July 24, 1994, p. 5.

7. William J. Donnelly and Daniel J. Brauner, "Why SOAP Is Bad for the Medical Record," *Archives of Internal Medicine* 152 (1992), 481–84. The subjectivity of the physician's observation started Alvan Feinstein on his quest; see the preface to his *Clinical Judgment* (Huntington, N.Y.: Krieger, 1967).

8. Simon S. Leopold, *The Principles and Methods of Physical Diagnosis: Correlation of Physical Signs with Certain Physiological and Pathological Changes in Disease,* 2nd ed. (Philadelphia: Saunders, 1957), p. 9.

9. The Atchley-Loeb Form—still so labeled—continues in use at Columbia University (Rita Charon, personal communication).

10. In *The Clinical Approach to the Patient* (Philadelphia: Saunders, 1969), which introduced psychosocial concerns into the clinical encounter, William L. Morgan and George L. Engel nevertheless omit the "chief complaint" without comment. Eric Cassell provocatively describes it as "valueless" and misleading and urges clarifying followup questions; see " 'Tell Me the Story of This Illness, Please,' " in *Talking with Patients* (Cambridge, Mass.: MIT Press, 1985), vol. 2, *Clinical Technique,* pp. 1–40, esp. p. 31.

11. Exacerbations of chronic disease are the exception. Such a case is usually written up as "carries a diagnosis of COPD" or "with a history of breast cancer," promoting this detail from the "past medical history" to an aspect of today's presentation.

12. Jules Cohen, personal communication.

13. Eric Cassell, *Talking with Patients*, especially vol. 2: *Clinical Technique*, pp. 157–61.

14. Morgan and Engel emphasize completeness and its usefulness in *Clinical Approach to the Patient*, pp. 56–58. More recent texts point out that a list of general questions may suffice; see Lynn S. Bickley and P. G. Szilagyi, *Bates' Guide to Physical Examination and History Taking*, 8th ed. (Philadelphia: Lippincott Williams and Wilkins, 2003), p. 3. Elizabeth Naumberg is the primary author of the chapter on interviewing and history-taking.

15. Michael Balint's classic account of the clinical "flash" predates this recent interest; see *The Doctor, His Patient, and the Illness* (New York: International University Press, 1957). William Carlos Williams's story "A Face of Stone" and many of the adventures of Sherlock Holmes provide narrative accounts of intuition. Anne Hunsaker Hawkins describes the imaginative insight gained from literature in "Medical Ethics and the Epiphanic Dimension of Narrative," in *Stories and Their Limits: Narrative Approaches to Bioethics*, ed. Hilde Lindemann Nelson (Routledge, 1997), pp. 153–70.

16. Georges Bordage and Madeleine Lemieux, "Semantic Structures and Diagnostic Thinking of Experts and Novices," *Academic Medicine* 66 (1990), S70–S72.

17. Faith Fitzgerald and Lawrence M. Tierney, Jr., "The Bedside Sherlock Holmes," *Western Journal of Medicine* 137 (1982), 169–75. Richard Selzer's story "Fairview" springs from a physician's observation of items on a patient's nightstand; see *Rituals of Surgery* (New York: Touchstone, 1974), pp. 29–36.

18. Patricia Benner, *From Novice to Expert: Excellence and Power in Clinical Nursing Practice* (Reading, Mass.: Addison-Wesley, 1984).

19. Jerome Kassirer and G. Anthony Gorry, "Clinical Problem Solving: A Behavioral Analysis," *Annals of Internal Medicine* 89 (1978), 245–55.

20. The monthly "Clinical Problem Solving" case instituted by Jerome Kassirer in the *New England Journal of Medicine* models early hypothesis-formation. See also Bickley and Szilagyi, *Bates' Guide*: "As you learn about the patient's story and the symptoms, you should be generating hypotheses about what body systems might be involved" (9).

21. Raymond H. Curry and Gregory Makoul, "An Active Learning Approach to Basic Clinical Skills," *Academic Medicine* 71 (1996), 33–36.

22. Perri Klass, "Classroom Ethics on the Job," *Harvard Medical Alumni Bulletin* 60 (1986), 36.

23. W. Scott Richardson and Douglas R. Reifler supplied these examples.

24. Sherlock Holmes's handling of an anomalous bit of information mirrors medicine's practical reasoning. There are two examples, and, not surprisingly, they contradict one another. In "The Six Napoleons," Inspector Lestrade puzzles over the villain's habit of breaking the valuable busts of Napoleon he has gone to great effort to steal: "Well, Mr. Holmes," he inquires, "what are we to do with that fact?" Holmes answers promptly, "To remember it—to docket it. We may come upon something later which will bear upon it." This is not negligence but a thoroughness that allows a judicious application of the tincture of time. But in "A Study in Scarlet," when an unexpectedly inert handrolled pill does not fit the hypothesis he has developed about the murderer's use of poison, anomaly provokes a different response:

"Surely my whole chain of reasoning cannot have been false. It is impossible! And yet this wretched dog is none the worse. Ah, I have it! I have it!" . . . Sherlock Holmes drew a long breath, and wiped the perspiration from his forehead. "I should have more faith," he said; "I ought to know by this time that when a fact appears to be opposed to a long train of deductions, it invariably proves to be capable of bearing some other interpretation"

This is a contradiction only when the two rules are taken out of their narrative contexts. The refusal to interpret that Sherlock Holmes finds practical early in an investigation makes little sense near the end.

25. James W. Mold and Howard F. Stein, "Sounding Board: The Cascade Effect in the Clinical Care of Patients," *New England Journal of Medicine* 314 (1986), 512–14.

26. Samuel Shem, *The House of God* (New York: Richard Marek, 1978), p. 376. The thirteenth law itself comes close to being a self-contained paradox, since its escape clause, "as much . . . as possible," is open to widely differing interpretations, some of which could countermand the nihilistic ideal. The Fat Man's "laws" are, of course, satiric maxims invented to counter those of his elders, especially the Chief of Medicine's belief that physicians should always do everything for every patient forever (257).

27. Willie Sutton's autobiography has recently been reprinted: Willie Sutton and Edward Linn, *Where the Money Was: Memoirs of a Bank Robber,* ed. Luc Sante (New York: Broadway Books, 2004).

28. William of Ockham, "Pluralitas non est ponenda sine necessitate."

29. W. T. Miller, "Occam versus Hickam," *Seminars in Roentgenology* 33 (1998), 213. I'm indebted to Alan M. Johnson for this reference.

30. An alternative to Hickam's dictum is discussed in Anthony A. Hilliard, Stefen E. Weinberger, Lawrence M. Tierney, Jr., David E. Midthun, and Sanjay Saint, "Occam's Razor versus Saint's Triad," *New England Journal of Medicine* 350 (2004), 599–603. Their fine case-based account of diagnostic tension ends with: "in patient care we cannot embrace either principle exclusively." I'm grateful to Mark Haupt for pointing out this article.

31. Mark E. Williams and N. M. Hadler, "Sounding Board: The Illness as the Focus of Geriatric Medicine," *New England Journal of Medicine* 308 (1983), 1357–60.

32. Jill A. Rhymes, Cheryl Woodson, Rochelle Sprage-Sachs, and Christine K. Cassel describe the collapse of family care arrangements after a diagnosis of tertiary syphilis in "Nonmedical Complications of Diagnostic Workup for Dementia," *Journal of the American Geriatric Society* 37 (1989), 1157–64.

33. Albert Jonsen and Stephen Toulmin, *The Abuses of Casuistry: A History of Moral Reasoning* (Berkeley: University of California, 1988), p. 257, pp. 252–53. Pellegrino and Thomasma distinguish the method of casuistry from the virtue of phronesis but grant that case-based reasoning calls for practical judgment in *The Virtues in Medical Practice* (New York: Oxford University Press, 1993), p. 85. See also Wayne C. Booth, *The Company We Keep: An Ethics of Fiction* (Berkeley: University of California Press, 1988).

34. The importance of time in the use of conflicting maxims is underscored by another pair of Sherlock Holmes's counterweighted pronouncements. On the way to the scene of the crime in the first of the stories, "A Study in Scarlet," Watson

asks why Holmes seems to be giving no thought to the problem. " 'No data yet,' he answered. 'It is a capital mistake to theorize before you have all the evidence. It biases the judgment.' " Soon, however, after favoring two dumbfounded Scotland Yard inspectors with a copiously detailed description of the murderer ("There's no room for mistake"), Holmes sets out with Watson to interview the policeman who discovered the body: " 'There is nothing like first-hand evidence,' he said. 'As a matter of fact my mind is entirely made up upon the case, but still we may as well learn all that is to be learned.' " Holmes never reconciles these two remarks, nor does Doyle give us any hint that either character regards them as in any way contradictory. They are situational rules, and, when used sequentially, their apparent conflict is overcome by the changing demands of the unfolding case.

Chapter 8

A version of this chapter was published as " 'Don't Think Zebras': Uncertainty, Interpretation, and the Place of Paradox in Clinical Education," *Theoretical Medicine* 5 (1996), 1–17. Along with an early version of chapter 7, parts of this chapter were presented to the University of Chicago's Case-Based Reasoning Group in the Department of Computer Science and to the University of North Carolina–Duke University Medical Ethics Group.

1. The distinction between technical and practical rationality is made by Donald A. Schön in *Educating the Reflective Practitioner: Toward a Design for Teaching and Learning in the Professions* (San Francisco: Jossey-Bass, 1987).

2. Clifford Geertz, describing the "immethodicalness" of commonsense "vernacular wisdom," cites contradictory proverbs in "Commonsense as a Cultural System," in *Local Knowledge: Further Essays in Interpretive Anthropology* (New York: Basic Books, 1983), p. 90.

3. Joseph Margolis, summary comments, Literature, Medicine, and Ethics Conference, East Carolina University School of Medicine, Greenville, N.C., April 1986. According to Chris Argyris and Donald A. Schön, this lack is characteristic of the professions, especially those that claim a technical rationality; see "Issues in Professional Education," in *Theory in Practice: Increasing Professional Effectiveness*, 2nd ed. (San Francisco: Jossey-Bass 1992), pp. 139–55.

4. Perri Klass, "Camels, Zebras, and Fascinomas," in *A Not Entirely Benign Procedure: Four Years as a Medical Student* (New York: Plume, 1994 [1987]), pp. 67–72.

5. Francis L. Brancati, "The Art of Pimping," *Journal of the American Medical Association* 262 (1989), 89–90. The American College of Physicians publishes a set of "Zebra Cards" to fit the pocket of the anxious learner.

6. The nature and corrigiblity of clinical judgment is often debated. Even the GPEP report took both sides; see Association of American Medical Colleges, *Physicians for the Twenty-First Century*: The GPEP Report (Washington, D.C.: Association of American Medical Colleges, 1984), no. 1, part 2. Clinical judgment is unteachable

only in that it cannot be taught as the "basic" sciences are taught, in lectures filled with memorizable facts delivered by a parade of experts who are seldom seen again. In actuality, "unreformed" clinical education has been fairly well designed to enable new physicians to observe the exercise of clinical judgment and to begin under supervision to exercise and take responsibility for their own.

7. Aristotle, *Nicomachean Ethics* 2.2, 1104a7. See also 6.5–8, especially 1141b8–1142a30.

8. Nicholas Christakis, *Death Foretold: Prophecy and Prognosis in Medical Care* (Chicago: University of Chicago Press, 1999).

9. It is difficult to describe so vital a rule as trivial, but it comes close: to live, all human beings need respiration and circulation. And, like legislative law, even this rule is revisable: trauma experts are now arguing that the standard ABCs of responding to a patient who is not breathing—clear the Airway, restart Breathing, maintain Circulation—should actually be ACB: mouth-to-mouth resuscitation is less important than chest compression. See Alfred Hallstrom, Leonard Cobb, Elsie Johnson, and Michael Copass, "Cardiopulmonary Resuscitation by Chest Compressions Alone or with Mouth to Mouth Ventilation," *New England Journal of Medicine* 342 (2000), 1546–53. I'm indebted to Kristi Kirschner for this reference.

10. David L. Sackett, Sharon E. Straus, W. Scott Richardson, William Rosenberg, and R. Brian Haynes, *Evidence Based Medicine*, 2nd ed. (New York: Churchill Livingstone, 2000), p. 30.

11. See Patricia Benner, *From Novice to Expert: Excellence and Power in Clinical Nursing Practice* (Reading, Mass.: Addison-Wesley, 1984), and Georges Bordage and Madeleine Lemieux, "Semantic Structures and Diagnostic Thinking of Experts and Novices," *Academic Medicine* 66 (1990), S70-S72.

12. A. Grant, N. O'Brien, and J. Marie-Theriese, "Cerebral Palsy among Children Born during the Dublin Randomized Trial of Intrapartum Monitoring," *Lancet* 334 (1989), 1233–36; and Jeffrey M. Perlman, "Review Article: Intrapartum Hypoxic-Ischemic Cerebral Injury and Subsequent Cerebral Palsy: Medicolegal Issues," *Pediatrics* 99 (1997), 851–59. Debate over EFM continues; see Renato Natale and Nancy Dodman, "Birth Can Be a Hazardous Journey: Electronic Fetal Monitoring Does Not Help," *Journal of Obstetrics and Gynaecology Canada* 23 (2003), 1007–9, which critiques the Society of Obstetrics and Gynaecology of Canada's slight concession to fetal monitoring use in its clinical practice guidelines. Thanks to Jeff Nisker.

13. Jerome Groopman, "Annals of Medicine: Second Opinion," *New Yorker*, January 24, 2000, pp. 40–49.

14. Samuel Shem, *The House of God* (New York: Richard Marek: 1978), p. 257.

15. The Cochrane Collaboration's database of systematic reviews is available online at cochrane.org/reviews/ (accessed April 28, 2005); the ACP Journal Club is available online at acpjc.org (accessed April 28, 2005).

16. Ross J. Simpson and Thomas R. Griggs, "Case Reports and Medical Progress," *Perspectives in Biology and Medicine* 28 (1985), 402–6; and Kathryn Montgomery Hunter, "'There Was This One Guy': The Uses of Anecdotes in Medicine," *Perspectives in Biology and Medicine* 29 (1986), 619–30.

17. Sackett et al., *Evidence Based Medicine*, pp. 13–27.

18. Geoffrey R. Norman, "The Non-Analytical Basis of Clinical Reasoning," presented to the Case-Based Reasoning Group in the Department of Computer Science, University of Chicago, December 14, 1994. See also H. G. Schmidt, G. R. Norman, and H.P.A. Boshuizen, "A Cognitive Perspective on Medical Expertise," *Academic Medicine* 65 (1990), 611–21; and Roger C. Schank, *Tell Me a Story: A New Look at Real and Artificial Memory* (New York: Scribner's, 1990).

19. C. S. Peirce, "Abduction and Induction," in *Philosophical Writings of Peirce*, ed. Justus Buchler (New York: Dover, 1955). See also Umberto Eco and Thomas A. Sebeok, eds., *The Sign of The Three: Dupin, Holmes, Peirce* (Bloomington: Indiana University Press, 1983).

20. Arthur E. Elstein, Gerald B. Holzman, Michael M. Ravitch, William A. Metheny, Margaret M. Holmes, Ruth B. Hoppe, Marilyn L. Rothert, and David R. Rovner, "Comparisons of Physician' Decisions Regarding Estrogen Replacement Therapy for Menopausal Women and Decisions Derived from a Decision Analytic Model," *American Journal of Medicine* 80 (1986), 246–58. Patient preference had a role in the relatively slow acceptance of HRT, but, given the encouraging data at the time, medical persuasion, if it had been exercised, would surely have encouraged greater use.

21. William A. Knaus, Douglas P. Wagner, and Joanne Lynn, "Short Term Mortality Predictions for Critically Ill Hospitalized Adults: Science and Ethics," *Science* 254 (1991), 389–94. See also Robert Zussman, *Intensive Care: Medical Ethics and the Medical Profession* (Chicago: University of Chicago Press, 1992).

22. Atul Gawande's title improves on Lewis Thomas's: *Complications: A Surgeon's Notes on an Imperfect Science* (New York: Metropolitan, 2002).

23. See Hans-Georg Gadamer, *The Enigma of Health: The Art of Healing in a Scientific Age*, trans. Jason Gaiger and Nicholas Walker (Stanford: Stanford University Press, 1996), p. 4.

24. Donald A. Schön, *Educating the Reflective Practitioner: Toward a New Design for Teaching and Learning in the Professions* (San Francisco: Jossey-Bass, 1987), p. 26.

25. Pierre Bourdieu, *The Logic of Practice*, trans. Richard Nice (Stanford: Stanford University Press, 1990), pp. 26, 91.

26. Stuart E. Dreyfus and Hubert L. Dreyfus, "A Five-Stage Model of the Mental Activities Involved in Directed Skill Acquisition," unpublished report to the U.S. Air Force Office of Scientific Research, Contract F49620-79-C-0063 (Berkeley: University of California at Berkeley, 1984); and Patricia Benner, *From Novice to Expert*.

27. Clifford Geertz, "Thick Description: Toward an Interpretive Theory of Culture," *The Interpretation of Cultures* (New York: Basic Books, 1973), pp. 28–29.

Chapter 9

The Northwestern firms had as their chiefs John Clarke, Murray Levin, James Webster, and then Warren Wallace. I'm grateful to them, to John Butter and Vinky Chadha, among others, who succeeded them, and to Lewis Landsberg, who began it all.

1. The seminar is described in Kathryn Montgomery, "Sherlock Holmes and Clinical Judgment," in *Teaching Literature and Medicine*, ed. Anne Hunsaker Hawkins and Marilyn Chandler McEntyre (New York: Modern Language Association, 1999), pp. 299–305. For the seminars generally, see James F. Bresnahan and Kathryn Montgomery Hunter, "Ethics Education at Northwestern University Medical School," *Academic Medicine*, 64 (1989), 740–43, and Kathryn Montgomery, Tod Chambers, and Douglas R. Reifler, "Medical Humanities Education at Northwestern University's Feinberg School of Medicine," *Academic Medicine* 78 (2003), 958–62.

2. David M. Waggoner, J. Dermot Frengley, Robert C. Griggs, and Charles H. Rammelkamp, "A 'Firm' System for Graduate Training in General Internal Medicine," *Journal of Medical Education* 54 (1979), 556–61. Thanks to Ray Curry for this reference.

3. Paul B. Beeson, "Some Good Features of the British National Health Services," *Journal of Medical Education* 49 (1974), 43–49. I'm grateful to Lewis Landsberg for his account of firms at the Beth Israel Hospital.

4. Jack Haas and William Shaffir describe the importance of self-presentation for the process of professionalization in "The Professionalization of Medical Students: Developing Competence and a Cloak of Competence," *Symbolic Interaction* 1 (1977), 71–88. All studies of self-presentation owe a debt to Erving Goffman, who described it as essential to establishing one's place in the social order in *The Presentation of Self in Everyday Life* (Garden City, N.Y.: Doubleday, 1959).

5. The characteristics, including seating patterns, of voluntary gatherings that make up a moral community have been described by Mitchell Duneier in his masterly *Slim's Table: Race, Respectability, and Masculinity* (Chicago: University of Chicago Press, 1992); see especially "Openness," pp. 86–92.

6. Charles Bosk, *Forgive and Remember: Managing Medical Failure* (Chicago: University of Chicago Press, 1979).

7. The exception to the even distribution of subspecialties was the assignment for several years of most geriatricians to the North Firm, while their division head was firm chief.

8. Coats independently owned were replaced by coats from the general hospital supply so that newness was noticeable only in coats of an unusual size. I am indebted for this observation to Maureen Brady Moran.

9. Like other rules in clinical practice, these are "bottom-up" rules, generated from observational experience and not deduced from theory or laws. Hence their practical force and their lack of codification. On the nature of such intermediate rules, see chapter 8.

10. The phrase *areas of unconformity* is borrowed from the geology of the Grand Canyon, with thanks to Julia E. Connelly.

11. Deans might sit there too. On one occasion, a retired chief of medicine, attending the East Firm by invitation, sat in the front row but near the window, and he turned his chair sideways, half facing the room.

12. William S. Gilbert and Arthur S. Sullivan, *The Mikado*, 1885, act I, with an echo of John Milton's assembly of fallen angels in *Paradise Lost*.

13. For a fascinating illustration of the "language" of visual symbols, see the semiotic system E. H. Gombrich constructed from all-but-identical British postage stamps in "Expresssion and Communication," *Meditations on a Hobby-Horse and Other Essays on the Theory of Art* [1963] (New York: Phaidon Press, 1994), pp. 56–69.

14. Residents and students soon learned to anticipate diagnostic categories by recognizing the subspecialists whom the firm chiefs had specifically invited to attend or, as with the psychiatrist in the North Firm, by their choice of seat.

15. This contrasts with the custom in surgery, where the first question about the care of trauma patients regularly falls to students, who answer, "Airway, Breathing, Circulation."

16. Donald O. Nutter suggested this further study.

17. Charles Bosk describes this process in *Forgive and Remember*. All students of medical education are indebted to Renée Fox, "Training for Uncertainty," in *The Student-Physician*, ed. Robert K. Merton, George Reader, and Patricia Kendall (Cambridge, Mass.: Harvard University Press, 1957), pp. 207–41.

18. Frederic W. Hafferty, "Beyond Curriculum Reform: Confronting Medicine's Hidden Curriculum," *Academic Medicine* 73 (1998), 403–7.

19. Or, as a student said (with appropriate minimization) about his calm, capable performance during the second week of his third year when the case he presented came under a senior faculty member's withering scrutiny: "You just have to show them you're a stand-up kind of guy."

Chapter 10

Early versions of this chapter were presented in 2001 at Penn State University Hershey Medical Center and to the members of the University of Bergen's Faculty Group on Health and Disease in a Cultural Perspective. I'm grateful to Anne Hunsaker Hawkins, Kirsti Malterud, Kari Tove Elvbakken, and Janeke Thiessen for their hospitality.

1. See references to the work of Patricia Benner, Stuart Dreyfus, and Georges Bordage for the forgetting that seems to be a part of the acquisition of expertise. The dehumanizing process has been well described in numerous autobiographical accounts of medical school; several are listed in the notes to the introduction.

2. See Frederic Hafferty, *Into the Valley: Death and the Socialization of Medical Students* (New Haven: Yale University Press, 1991); and Douglas R. Reifler, " 'I Actually Don't Mind the Bone Saw': Narratives of Gross Anatomy," *Literature and Medicine* 15 (1996), 183–99.

3. Donald A. Schön describes this "naming and framing" as a part of "knowing-in-action" in his study of the epistemology of practice: *Educating the Reflective Practitioner* (San Francisco: Jossey-Bass, 1987), pp. 4–5.

4. Emile Durkheim, *Professional Ethics and Civic Morals*, trans. Cornelia Brookfield (London: Routledge and Kegan Paul, 1957), pp. 4–5.

5. Katie Watson points out that the phrase is also the opening line of a joke—"A skeleton walks into a bar . . ." (personal communication). Its echo gives the clinical story a touch of the outrageously unexpected, the noncanonical.

6. Emmanuel Levinas, "Ethics as First Philosophy," trans. Seán Hand and Michael Temple, in *The Levinas Reader*, ed. Seán Hand (Oxford: Blackwell, 1989), pp. 75–87.

7. Benjamin Tucker, "An Apology on Biko," *New York Times* October 25, 1991. The full text of the letter, addressed to the South African Medical and Dental Council, originally appeared in the daily newspaper the *Sowetan*.

8. Charles Bosk, *Forgive and Remember: Managing Medical Failure* (Chicago: University of Chicago Press, 1979).

9. Pedro Laín Entralgo, *The Therapy of the Word in Classical Antiquity*, ed. and trans. L. J. Rather and John M. Sharp (New Haven: Yale University Press, 1970), and Michel Foucault, *The Birth of the Clinic: An Archeology of Medical Perception*, trans. A. M. Sheridan Smith (New York: Vintage, 1975).

10. Karl Marx, *The Eighteenth Brumaire of Louis Bonaparte*, 1851–52, chap. 1.

11. John Dewey, *Human Nature and Conduct: An Introduction to Social Psychology* (1922), in *The Middle Works, 1899–1924*, vol. 14 (Carbondale: Southern Illinois State University Press, 1988), p. 15.

12. For exploration of these questions in other fields, see, for example, Harold Bloom, *The Anxiety of Influence: A Theory of Poetry*, 2nd ed. (New York: Oxford University Press, 1997), and Carlo Ginzburg, *The Cheese and the Worms: The Cosmos of a Sixteenth-Century Miller*, trans. John and Anne Tedeschi (Baltimore: Johns Hopkins Press, 1980).

13. Pierre Bourdieu, *The Logic of Practice*, trans. Richard Nice (Stanford: Stanford University Press, 1990), pp. 57, 26, 61, 91.

14. Clifford Geertz, "Common Sense as a Cultural System," in *Local Knowledge: Further Essays in Interpretive Anthropology* (New York: Basic Books, 1983), pp. 75 and 84.

15. The Accreditation Council on Graduate Medical Education (ACGME) has embarked on just such a radical shift. Within a year that supervisory body both imposed an 80-hour work week on residency programs and asked them to devise ways of satisfying six new "competencies," all of which are arguably components of clinical judgment. See the ACGME web site, availabe online at: www.acgme.org (accessed May 4, 2004).

16. Charles Taylor, *Sources of the Self: The Making of the Modern Identity* (Cambridge, Mass.: Harvard University Press, 1989).

17. Library shelves are packed with studies of professionalization and how that process is accomplished, beginning with Everett Hughes, "The Study of Occupations," in *Sociology Today*, ed. R. K. Merton, L. Broom, and L. S. Cottrell, Jr. (New York: Basic Books, 1959).

18. Eric Cassell describes "medical training—particularly in the post-graduate years—[as] directed to the moral development of physicians, not only the technical," in *Nature of Suffering and the Goals of Medicine*, p. 75.

19. Hubert L. Dreyfus argues that emotional investment is necessary for the development of expertise in *On the Internet* (London: Routledge, 2001).

20. William L. Morgan, personal communication. Sherwin B. Nuland makes the same distinction in arguing for a broadened (and well-funded) medical education that includes the humanities; see "The Uncertain Art: The True Healers," *American Scholar,* spring 1999, pp. 125–28.

21. The introduction of the medical humanities in the curriculum has focused attention on the person who is becoming a physician; for example, Rita Charon's parallel chart concerns the patient but encourages the habit of more nuanced interpretation in her students. See Melanie Thernstrom, "The Writing Cure," *New York Times Magazine,* April 18, 2004, pp. 42–47.

22. Howard Becker, *Boys in White: Student Culture in Medical School* (Chicago: University of Chicago Press, 1961); Sinclair Lewis, *Arrowsmith* (New York: Grosset and Dunlap, 1925).

23. William Osler, "The Student Life," *Æquanimitas* (London: H. K. Lewis, 1904); Raymond H. Curry, "A Doctor in the House," Alpha Omega Alpha lecture, Chicago, November 12, 1999.

24. Myrtle Logan Pleune observed: "In my day residents couldn't be married. They still can't be, of course, but now they are allowed to try" (personal communication).

25. See Julia E. Connelly, "The Other Side of Professionalism: Doctor-to-Doctor," *Cambridge Quarterly of Healthcare Ethics* 12 (2003), 178–83, on the personal and professional price of self-sacrifice. There is a full discussion of professionalism in the *American Journal of Bioethics* (summer 2004), in response to Mark Kuczewski and Deleese Wear, "The Professionalism Movement: Can We Pause?" *American Journal of Bioethics* 4:2 (2004), 1–10.

26. This expectation supplies much of the shock of William Carlos Williams's story "A Face of Stone," when the physician-narrator refuses to go out on a winter night to see an immigrant couple and their baby. "My dear!"—a rare line of dialogue given to his wife—underlines the violation.

27. George Engel used this phrase often in conversation and in lectures at the University of Rochester in the 1980s; Alvan R. Feinstein gave his "clinimetrics" articles the title "An Additional Basic Science for Clinical Medicine, I–IV," *Annals of Internal Medicine* 99 (1983), 393–97, 554–60, 705–12, 843–48.

28. This careful scrutiny of clinical method might seem to prove that clinical medicine is moving from a practice to a science because it appears to challenge Bourdieu's assertion that practical knowledge characteristically "exclude[s] from the experience any inquiry as to its own conditions of possibility." But while this almost continual review subjects the acts and decisions of beginning physicians to the judgment of their teachers and peers, academic medicine does not call into question medicine's basic assumptions or its method—its "conditions of possibility." "Reflexive attention to action remains subordinate to the [practitioner's] pursuit of the result and to the search . . . for maximum effectiveness of the effort expended" (91).

29. Jerome P. Kassirer and Richard I. Kopelman, *Learning Clinical Reasoning* (Baltimore: Williams and Wilkins, 1991); see also the *New England Journal of Medicine's* monthly section "Clinical Problem Solving," which began July 1991, when Kassirer assumed editorship of the journal.

30. William J. Donnelly and Daniel J. Brauner, "Why SOAP Is Bad for the Medical Record," *Archives of Internal Medicine* 152 (1992), 481–84.

31. William Osler, "Æquanimitas [1905]," in *Æquanimitas*, 3rd ed. (New York: McGraw-Hill, 1932), pp. 1–12.

32. Samuel Shem, *The House of God* (New York: Richard Marek, 1973), p. 376.

33. "Somehow, this field observation became a normative prescription, and physicians for decades seemed to consider detachment a goal": Rita Charon, "Narrative Medicine: A Model for Empathy, Reflection, Profession, and Trust," *Journal of the American Medical Association* 286 (2001), 1899. See also Jodi Halpern, *From Detached Concern to Empathy: Humanizing Medical Practice* (New York: Oxford University Press, 2001).

34. David Reiser, "Struggling to Stay Human in Medicine: One Student's Reflections on Becoming a Doctor," *New Physician*, May 1973.

35. John Lantos, *The Lazarus Case: Life and Death Issues in Neonatal Care* (Baltimore: Johns Hopkins, 2001), pp. 50–51.

36. William Branch and Anthony Suchman, "Meaningful Experiences in Medicine," *American Journal of Medicine* 88 (1990), 56–59.

37. ABIM End-of-Life Patient Care Project, *Caring for the Dying: Identification and Promotion of Physician Competency: Personal Narratives* (Philadelphia: American Board of Internal Medicine, 1997). Thanks to Chris Cassell and Linda Blank for replacing the copy I gave away.

38. There is a long pre-Kantian tradition, including Augustine and David Hume, that regards emotion as part of rationality. Sidney Callahan argued for its inclusion in "The Role of Emotion in Ethical Decisionmaking, "*Hastings Center Report* 18 (June–July 1988), 9–14, as has Julia E. Connelly, "Emotions and Clinical Decisions," *Journal of General Internal Medicine* 13 (1990), 1. More recently the argument has been made by Martha Nussbaum at length in *Upheavals of Thought* (Cambridge: Cambridge University Press, 2002), and from a neurological standpoint by Antonio R. Damasio, *Descartes' Error: Emotion, Reason, and the Human Brain* (New York: Anchor Books, 1994).

39. Robert M. Veatch, "The Medical Model: Its Nature and Problems," *Hastings Center Studies* 1 (1973), 59–76. See also William F. May, *The Physician's Covenant: Images of the Healer in Medical Ethics* (Philadelphia: Westminster, 1983).

40. G. O. Gabbard and R. W. Menninger, "The Psychology of Postponement in the Medical Marriage," *Journal of the American Medical Association* 261 (1989), 2378–81. I'm grateful to Joel Frader for this reference.

Chapter 11

A version of this chapter was first presented November 15, 1996 at the sesquicentennial of the medical school at the State University of New York at Buffalo and was published in *Ethical Issues in Heath Care on the Frontiers of the Twentieth-Century*, vol. 65, Philosophy and Medicine, ed. James Bono and Steven Wear (Dordrect: Kluwer, 2000), pp. 205–19.

1. Charles E. Rosenberg, *The Care of Strangers: The Rise of America's Hospital System* (New York: Basic Books, 1987).

2. James F. Childress and Mark Siegler, "Metaphors and Models of Doctor-Patient Relationships: Their Implications for Autonomy," *Theoretical Medicine* 5 (1984), 17–30.

3. Robert M. Veatch, "Models for Ethical Medicine in a Revolutionary Age," *Hastings Center Report* 2 (1972), 5–7. William May, following Paul Ramsey, supplies another model in *The Physician's Covenant: Images of the Healer in Medical Ethics* (Philadelphia: Westminster, 1983).

4. Quoted in Pedro Laín Entralgo, *Doctor and Patient*, trans. Frances Partridge (New York: McGraw-Hill, 1969), p. 7. Laín's epigraph, of which I have quoted only the first quarter, is from Seneca's *De Beneficiis*, 6.16.

5. Aristotle, *Nicomachean Ethics*, trans. Terence Irwin (Indianapolis: Hackett, 1985) 8.3, 1156a20.

6. Which of Aristotle's criteria for friendship is met by this notion of therapy is arguable. See Robert Bellah, Richard Madsen, William M. Sullivan, Ann Swidler, and Steven M. Tipton, *Habits of the Heart: Individualism and Commitment in American Life* (Berkeley: University of California, 1985), p. 115–23. I'm grateful to Tod Chambers for reminding me of this study and for telling me about Paul Rabinow's struggle with the problem of friendship, described in *Reflections on Fieldwork in Morocco* (Berkeley: University of California Press, 1977), pp. 142–48.

7. Edmund D. Pellegrino and David C. Thomasma, *The Virtues in Medical Practice* (New York: Oxford University Press, 1993), pp. 82–83.

8. James F. Drane, "Character and the Moral Life: A Virtue Approach to Biomedical Ethics" in *A Matter of Principles? Ferment in U.S. Bioethics*, ed. Edward R. DuBose, R. P. Hamel, Lawrence J. O'Connell (Valley Forge, Pa.: Trinity Press International, 1994), pp. 284–309.

9. Rosamond Rhodes, "Love Thy Patient: Justice, Caring, and the Doctor-Patient Relationship, *Cambridge Quarterly of Healthcare and Bioethics* 4 (1995), 434–47.

10. M. Therese Lysaught, "Who Is My Neighbor?" *Second Opinion* 18 (October 1992), 59–67; David Hilfiker, "Clint Wooder," *Second Opinion* (October 1992), pp. 43–53.

11. Ezekiel J. Emanuel and Linda L. Emanuel, "Four Models of the Physician-Patient Relationship," *Journal of the American Medical Association* 267 (1992), 2221–26.

12. Chalmers Clark and Gerrit Kimsma, "Medical Friendships in Assisted Dying," *Cambridge Quarterly for Healthcare Ethics* 13 (2004), 61–68.

13. Francis W. Peabody, "The Care of the Patient," *Journal of the American Medical Association* 88 (1927), 877–82.

14. W. Eugene Smith, "Country Doctor," *Life*, 1948; collected in Gilles Mora, *W. Eugene Smith's Photographs, 1934–1975* (New York: Abrams, 1998), pp. 74–87.

15. Charles Fried, "The Lawyer as Friend: The Moral Foundations of the Lawyer-Client Relation," *Yale Law Review* 85 (1976), 1060–89.

16. The exceptions are medical ethicists, who to some degree are allied with the profession; they do not write as patients.

17. William T. Branch and Anthony Suchman, "Meaningful Experiences in Medicine," *American Journal of Medicine* 88 (1990), 56–59.

18. Edward L. Erde and Anne Hudson Jones, "Diminished Capacity, Friendship and Medical Paternalism: Two Case Studies from Fiction," *Theoretical Medicine* 4 (1983), 303–22.

19. P.M.L. Illingworth, "The Friendship Model of Physician/Patient Relationship and Patient Autonomy," *Bioethics* 2 (1988), 22–36. Her view was challenged by David N. James, who maintains that the trust essential to good patient-physician relationships resembles friendship closely enough to warrant the exploration of the model, "The Friendship Model: A Reply to Illingworth," *Bioethics* 3 (1989), 142–46.

20. Ann Folwell Stanford and Nancy M. P. King, "Patient Stories, Doctor Stories, and True Stories: A Cautionary Reading," *Literature and Medicine* 11 (1992), 185–99.

21. Michael T. Taussig, "Reification and the Consciousness of the Patient," *Social Science and Medicine* 143 (1980), 12; Arthur Kleinman, *The Illness Narratives: Suffering, Healing and the Human Condition* (New York: Basic Books, 1988).

22. I am indebted to Douglas R. Reifler for this observation.

23. Leo Tolstoy, "The Death of Ivan Ilych," in *The Death of Ivan Ilych and Other Stories*, trans. Aylmer Maude (New York: Signet, 1960), p. 121. Ivan Ilych is a "new man," a bureaucrat, at the time a decided advance over the bribable functionaries of the old regime.

24. Anne Hunsaker Hawkins, *Reconstructing Illness: Studies in Pathography*, 2nd ed. (West Lafayette, Ind.: Purdue University Press, 1999); Arthur Frank, "Reclaiming an Orphan Genre: First-Person Narratives of Illness," *Literature and Medicine* 13 (1994), 1–21.

25. Reynolds Price, *A Whole New Life: An Illness and a Healing* (New York: Athenaeum, 1994), p. 145.

26. Franz Ingelfinger, "Arrogance," *New England Journal of Medicine* 303 (1980), 1507–11; and see Edward E. Rosenbaum, *A Taste of My Own Medicine: When the Doctor Is the Patient* (New York: Random House, 1988). On the healing power of authority, see Eric Cassell, *The Healer's Art* (Cambridge, Mass.: MIT Press, 1985), and Sherwin Nuland, "The Uncertain Art: Mind, Body, and the Doctor," *American Scholar*, summer 2001, pp. 123–26.

27. Norman Cousins, *Anatomy of an Illness as Perceived by the Patient: Reflections on Healing and Regeneration* (New York: Norton, 1979).

28. W. H. Auden, "The Art of Healing: *In Memoriam David Protetch, MD*," in Richard Reynolds and John Stone, *On Doctoring: Stories, Poems, Essays* (New York: Simon and Schuster, 1991), pp. 168–70.

29. Anatole Broyard, *Intoxicated by My Illness* (New York: Clarkson Potter, 1992), p. 44; the emphasis is Broyard's.

30. Howard Brody, *Placebos and the Philosophy of Medicine: Clinical, Conceptual and Ethical Issues* (Chicago: University of Chicago Press, 1980). See also Nuland, "Uncertain Art."

31. John Berger, *A Fortunate Man*, with photographs by Jean Mohr (New York: Holt, 1967), p. 103. Mohr's photographs are a reminder that the subject of W. Eugene Smith's iconic photographs in *Country Doctor* is a neighbor rather than a friend.

32. John Stone, "He Makes a House Call," in *In All This Rain* (Baton Rouge: Louisiana State University Press, 1981), pp. 4–5.

33. The line "Something there is that does not love a wall" occurs as often as "Good fences make good neighbors"; Robert Frost, "Mending Wall," in *North of Boston* (New York: Holt, 1914).

34. Lyndon Baines Johnson, inaugural address, January 20, 1965.

35. Luke 10:29.

36. Paul Rabinow wrestles with the problem of friendship between the anthropologist and a member of the culture studied in *Reflections on Fieldwork in Morocco*, pp. 142–48.

37. The term is used by H. Tristram Engelhardt, Jr., in *The Foundations of Bioethics*, 2nd ed. (New York: Oxford University Press, 1996), pp. 6–7.

Chapter 12

Part of this chapter was included in "Information Is Not Enough," in *Ethical Decisions in Cancer Care*, ed. Peter Angelos (Dordrect: Kluwer, 1999), pp. 13–21. I am indebted to Julie Goldman, who brought an anthropologist's training and a patient's perspective to the National Comprehensive Cancer Center's communication task force. Her videotaped conversation with her doctor, an oncologist who had overridden her advance directive not long before, is a striking inquiry into the physician's clinical ethos. And I'm grateful to Sheila Rose Carrel, a survivor of breast cancer at 32 who shares two grandsons with me, for promising, "One day, when you least expect it, you'll be going down the road with the radio on and suddenly you'll hear the music again."

1. See Eric Cassell, *The Healer's Art* (New York: Penguin, 1976), and *The Nature of Suffering and the Goals of Medicine* (New York: Oxford University Press, 1991), and Howard Brody, " 'My Story Is Broken: Can You Help Me Fix It?': Medical Ethics and the Joint Construction of Narrative, *Literature and Medicine* 13 (1994), 79–92.

2. In the long term, however, improved health has been due to improved agriculture, clean water, better nutrition and hygiene, and good sewerage; see Thomas McKeown, *The Modern Rise of Population* (London: Edward Arnold, 1976), pp. 152–63.

3. See Joanne Trautmann [Banks], ed., *The Healing Arts in Dialogue: Medicine and Literature* (Carbondale: Southern Illinois University Press, 1981). This, however, is no argument against the validity of common experience or the authenticity of the experiencing self.

4. Nicholas A. Christakis, *Death Foretold: Prophecy and Prognosis in Medical Care* (Chicago: University of Chicago Press, 1999). Christakis is concerned with misprognosis at the end of life, while I am addressing prognostics at the time of diagnosis. Physicians' earlier, well-justified reluctance to specify limited survival time—for reasons Christakis's dedication to his mother poignantly illustrates—seems to have corrupted the tradition of prognosis when patients are close to death.

5. Marcus Conant quoted in Ronald Bayer and Gerald M. Oppenheimer, *AIDS Doctors: Voices from the Epidemic* (New York: Oxford University Press, 2000), pp. 157–60.

6. Peter Angelos, "Pattern of Physician-Patient Communication: Results of Preliminary Studies," presented to a symposium in honor of David L. Nahrwold, Northwestern University Medical School, February 27, 1998, Chicago.

7. This goes against the implicit recommendation of patient support groups.

8. Daniel Kahneman and Amos Tversky, "The Framing of Decisions and the Psychology of Choice," *Science* 211 (1981), 453–58. See also their earlier "Judgment under Uncertainty," *Science* 185 (1974), 1124–31. More recently, Herbert Simon's concept of bounded rationality has prompted researchers to make sense of habitual violations of logic; see also Gerd Gigerenzer, Peter M. Todd, and the ABC Research Group, *Simple Heuristics That Makes Us Smart* (New York: Oxford University Press, 1999).

9. Stephen Jay Gould, "The Median Is Not the Message," in *Narrative Based Medicine*, ed. Trisha Greenhalgh and Brian Hurwitz (London: British Medical Journal Press, 1999), pp. 31, 33.

10. Sidney T. Bogardus, Jr., Eric Holmboe, and James F. Jekel, "Perils, Pitfalls, and Possibilities in Talking about Medical Risk," *Journal of the American Medical Association* 281 (199), 1037–41.

11. Aristotle, *Metaphysics*, bk. 6.

12. Anatole Broyard's exemption of his surgeon in *Intoxicated by My Illness* is made partly because that frosty eminence had the good sense to have as his associate a physician who was willing to talk. Nevertheless, Broyard's wish that "my doctor would meditate on my illness for just five minutes," quoted on p. 184, is the most moving part of the book. Patricia Benner's comment was made at the International Bioethics Retreat, Cambridge, England, September 14, 2000.

13. Dewitt Stettin, Jr., "Coping with Blindness," *New England Journal of Medicine* 305 (1981), 458–60.

14. William Osler, *Æquinimitas and Other Essays* (London: H.K. Lewis, 1904).

15. Francis W. Peabody, "The Care of the Patient," *Journal of the American Medical Association* 88 (1927), 877–82.

16. See Eric Cassell, "The Principles of the Belmont Report Revisited: How Have Respect for Persons, Benevolence, and Justice Been Applied to Clinical Medicine?" *Hastings Center Report* 30 (July–August 2000), pp. 12–21.

17. Richard Schechner, *Between Theater and Anthropology* (Philadelphia: University of Pennsylvania Press, 1985), pp. 121–26. Thanks to Tod Chambers for this reference.

18. Victor Turner, *From Ritual to Theater* (New York: Performing Arts Journal Press), p. 93.

19. Claude Levi-Strauss, *Structural Anthropology* (New York: Basic Books, 1963), pp. 167–85; Schechner cites this skeptical shaman in *Between Theater and Anthropology*, pp. 121.

20. See Bill Moyers, *Healing and the Mind* (New York: Doubleday, 1993), based on the PBS series of the same title and shown the same year.

21. Reading this chapter, she wrote, "I wanted to make it more of a *transaction*—letting him know that I was agreeing to let him learn on me. . . . I felt I was giving him a chance to back out and if he didn't, then he could do it right."

22. Edmund D. Pellegrino, "The Metamorphosis of Medical Ethics: A Thirty-Year Retrospective," *Journal of the American Medical Association* 269 (1993), 1158–62.

23. Richard Rorty distinguishes ironists, who recognize the contingency of their knowledge and belief, from theologians and metaphysicians in Richard Rorty, *Contingency, Irony, Solidarity* (New York: Cambridge University Press, 1989). When I tried this idea out in conversation with Barry Saunders, a general internist with a Ph.D. in religious studies, he laughed: "It's worked for me!"

24. Pierre Bourdieu, *The Logic of Practice*, trans. Richard Nice (Stanford: Stanford University Press, 1990), p. 61.

25. Paul Auster, *Mr. Vertigo* (New York: Penguin, 1994), p. 137.

INDEX

⌒